CHEATING COVID

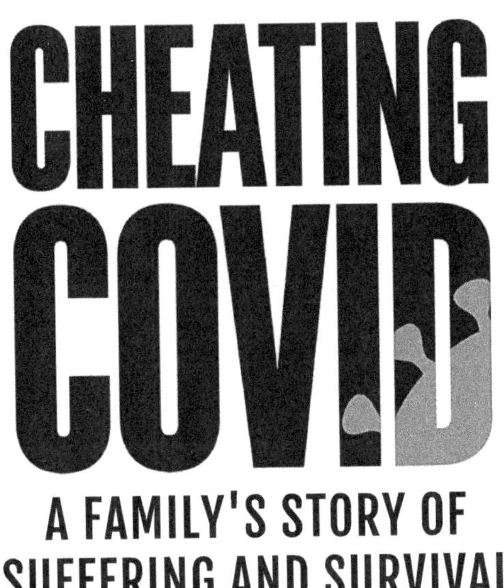

CHEATING COVID

A FAMILY'S STORY OF SUFFERING AND SURVIVAL

MANASI GOKHALE, ROHAN BAVADEKAR
AND SHARMISTHA CHAUDHURI

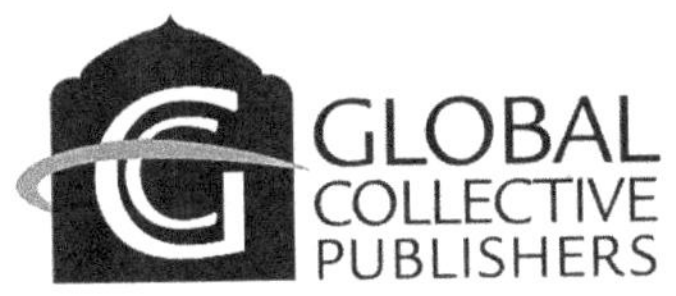

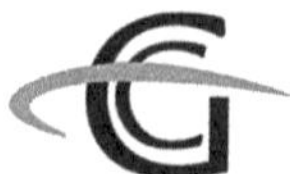

Published by Global Collective Publishers
16 North Bryn Mawr Ave., #1355
Bryn Mawr, PA 19010
U.S.A.
www.globalcollectivepublishers.com

First published in India by Vitasta Publishing Pvt Ltd

Paperback ISBN: 978-1-954021-91-4
eBook ISBN: 978-1-954021-92-1

Edited by Manjula Lal
Cover Photo by Manasi Gokhale & Rohan Bavadekar
Typeset & Cover Design by Somesh Kumar Mishra

To
All healthcare workers around
the world who are working
tirelessly to save lives

Contents

Foreword

The COVID-19 pandemic has changed our lives beyond belief and imagination. It is perhaps the first worldwide crisis everyone has faced together, knowingly or unknowingly. Nothing in life is to be feared; it is only to be understood. Now is the time to understand more so that we may fear less. Humanity is trying to cope with the stress and strain of the 'new normal' in its unique ways.

I perceive sharing experiences as one way to find a common thread in that rich though tragic human experience. Furthermore, there is no better way of communicating than writing a book or a novel. Here in this book that you are about to read, the authors share an intensely personal experience during the pandemic. It is narrated as a story that unites as a shared human experience—how the husband survived the complications of the coronavirus infection, and how his partner fought from behind the scenes, anxiously. This is their story; and they share their experiences candidly.

When I was asked to write a foreword for this story,

I wondered, 'What is my qualification?' But as I read the manuscript, I began to feel that I am one of the narrative characters. Factually, I am a small part of the story but only from a distance.

A friend of mine asked me to help assess his friend's situation admitted to a peripheral hospital in Houston, Texas, with COVID-19 infection. 'He's not doing well' is how my friend put it. Having worked at the Baylor College of Medicine, Houston for the last thirty-two years, and as Chief of Pulmonary, Critical Care Medicine for over fifteen of these years, I know most Intensive Care doctors in the United States of America (USA) as former trainees or colleagues. I spoke to the physician taking care of the patient, who happened to be one of my erstwhile trainees. He confirmed what I had thought, that the patient indeed had Covid Acute Respiratory Distress Syndrome (ARDS). The patient had suffered lung and kidney failures, was on a ventilator and receiving dialysis. The physician felt the patient needed a higher level of care, including ECMO (supplies oxygen to the body by the help of an external machine to unload the heart and lungs). However, due to the involvement of multiple organs and other complications, one other hospital did not feel the transfer was possible. No, the patient was definitely not doing well.

Confusion and despair became the order of the day in the life of the patient's wife. I called to explain the situation, and the risks involved in transferring such a sick patient to our medical college hospital.

First, the transfer process itself is risky for sick and unstable patients (Rohan, the patient, was on very high settings on the ventilator plus the many lifesaving drug infusions). Second, there are many steps involved in transfers (disconnecting the monitors; reconnecting to portable ventilator, heart monitor, pressure monitor then moving on to the stretcher; roll the stretcher with all the temporary monitoring devices; and transport ventilator to the helicopter or ambulance). Any step can go wrong during transport. Then, the entire process has to be reversed at the receiving hospital.

Hospitals do these steps every day, but the process itself is fraught with risk of either the underlying medical condition getting worse and/or missteps. In my experience, there is always an increase in the heart rates of the caring team during this entire process no matter how many times one has done it. In Rohan's case, my fear was the family not understanding the severe risks involved in the process.

Rohan's wife, Manasi, readily agreed to the transfer. So, I initiated the process and Rohan was transferred by air to one of our hospitals in the Texas Medical Center.

The book describes in vivid detail the rollercoaster ride of Rohan's hospitalisation. COVID-19 patients in the ICUs are uniquely different from other ICU patients. They have virtually no personal contact with their near and dear ones. To this, add the impact of good-intentioned-but-unsolicited advice from relatives and friends. It is an unmitigated chaos.

I very much enjoyed the manuscript. It is an intensely-personal account where even mundane events become exciting page-turners. The trans-continental family dialogues, anxious moments of the elderly parents of the main characters take us back to our own trials and tribulations and add a new perspective to life. Manasi comes across as a strong-willed woman facing adversity with fortitude and courage.

I quote one sentence from the book that tells it all: 'Eight minutes. Only eight minutes of flying time that could be the deciding factor between life and death. However, was it even possible to fly'. This line encapsulates the story of ordinary people surmounting extraordinary situations with faith, courage, and more importantly, grace.

Rohan displayed extraordinary patience and courage going through complex and often unpleasant procedures with faith and determination. The prolonged rehabilitation he needed and the attendant cognitive problems are not easy to handle.

The book is very interesting as it captures the patient's perspective and the family struggles put in the backdrop of the rapidly-changing medical scenario. This book validates the extensive research done around not only the patient but also the much-less recognised family struggles. The psychological toll on the family has only been recognised, even by the medical profession, in the last decade or so.

This book will serve as an eye-opener to the medical

profession while validating the feelings of the many families devastated by critical illness. I would venture to say that families and patient survivors of critical illness will feel vindicated as they go through the complicated course of hope, desperation, helplessness, and denial—a common experience of jumbled emotions.

Many patients with prolonged critical illness develop anxiety, depression and post-traumatic stress disorder (PTSD). Spousal support and empathy are crucial for recovery. Rohan was fortunate in receiving such support in abundance. However, in the end, Rohan comes across as a true survivor. We are seeing this in the post-COVID clinic very clearly.

What is also less recognised in public is the impact of critical illness on a family. This has been exaggerated in the somewhat cruel realities of the COVID-19 pandemic—the isolation, the strict no-visitation policy even when the loved one is dying or has passed away, the overstretched health care personnel who may not be able to give the time to update the family, loss of income, loss of insurance, mounting medical bills, and uncertainty of outcome despite the tough fight. They all contribute to exaggerate the situation. A third of the families of critically-ill patients also suffer from anxiety, depression and PTSD. They need to take care of themselves too before it affects the rest of the family.

Talking to Manasi, I advised her on dealing with good-natured but uninformed advice from friends and relatives. In my over four-decade experience treating patients in ICUs, I find that the most crucial stumbling block for a realistic understanding of the patient's situation by the spouse and/or children is the confusion created by well-wishers. Please read the book, and you will understand how important it is.

Another source of false hopes or despair about diseases and treatments is the web. The internet is an excellent source of information. However, one must be cautious. Most do not read scientific articles full of empirical jargon. Instead, they read the eye-catching titles only. I would advise to always remember the internet is an open-architecture forum and anyone can publish anything. The story you are about to read illustrates this point very well. It is not easy to be a patient, but it is harder to be a significant other. I know it is easier said than done, but we must learn to accept life on life's terms.

This co-written book takes us back to the early phase of the current pandemic. It was a journey set in the middle of many uncertainties, false hopes, and social turmoil. It is a story of selfless service of medical personnel, dutiful near and dear of thankful patients balancing and surviving a range of emotions. 'The best and most beautiful things in the world cannot be seen or even touched. They must be felt with the heart,' said Helen Keller. I am sure this book will touch your heart.

—Kalpalatha K Guntupalli
MD, FCCM, Master FCCP, MACP
Frances K Friedman and Oscar Friedman, MD '36.
Endowed Professor for Pulmonary Disorders,
Ben Taub General Hospital
Program Director, Critical Care Fellowship,
Department of Medicine, Baylor College of Medicine

Prologue

28 March 2020

Eight minutes. Only eight minutes of flying time that could be the deciding factor between life and death. However, was it even possible to fly?

I was intubated, incommunicative, critical, my kidney failing every minute. Lying on a dreary bed, hooked up to tubes, I was fighting to stave off the novel Coronavirus symptoms that were spreading through my body, wrecking me from within. Like troops attacking an intruder, my immune system was attacking the virus, but here's the tricky thing—the immune system attacks the pathogens but the side-effects can be devastating. My chest x-rays showed no hope, my resting heart rate had shot up to 160 and an arterial line had been placed the night before to monitor my fluctuating blood pressure. It had been four days since the ambulance ride from home to the nearby emergency room, and then to a smaller hospital in Texas' largest metropolis, which had provisions for virus-infected patients.

Coronavirus was still in its nascent stages in the USA, the country still unsure of how deadly this virus strain could be. How fast it could strike down its people, with deaths reaching record numbers. There were growing cases, of course; the first case of the novel virus was recorded in January, two months ago, in a Washington state patient who flew back from Wuhan, China, the epicentre of it all. By early February, non-travel related cases of the virus were reported in the news. Yet, it seemed to me, people were still not taking it seriously.

My wife, Manasi, too, had contracted the virus. She was at home with our three children, who were showing symptoms as well. Completely home-bound, unwell, coughing, delirious, Manasi didn't care about her situation. I don't think she realised the severity of her state; her sole focus at that point was to get me a fighting chance to survive. And that would come with an ECMO (extracorporeal membrane oxygenation) treatment which was not available where I was admitted.

'Everything we are trying is going in the opposite direction. CPR is not advisable,' a hospital doctor explained to Manasi, giving her facts about my deteriorating health.

'I don't care. You will administer CPR to Rohan as many times as required,' she said, furious at the thought that I wasn't getting help, and battling her own sickness with Gatorade, trying to stay hydrated, and medication.

My sudden renal failure and the need for partial dialysis had put off the hospital in trying to secure my

ECMO treatment in the nearby top-notch hospital, an internationally-recognised leader in medical research and innovation*. Just eight minutes away.

'It will be of no help to Rohan,' repeated naysayers.

It would mean moving me in my unstable condition. It could be fatal, I could die right then. No medical institute wants blood on their hands.

Manasi didn't care. Over a morning video call, she had seen me: my ventilator-dependent vegetative state, with only my privates modestly covered. Doctors tried to explain the futility of what she was attempting—moving me eight minutes away in a chopper when even a slight touch by the staff was destabilising my vitals.

My brother-in-law, Bhushan, who lived three hours away in Austin, had driven down in the morning to be outside our house. To be there for his sister, whom he loved more than life. 'Can the ECMO machine be brought to Rohan?' he asked Manasi, conversing with her from the yard. That possibility was ruled out quickly when he realised what exactly the machine did: providing heart and lung support to the grievously injured or after surgery when one's organs need to recover and heal.

'You are making a mistake,' the cardiology specialist warned. 'ECMO will not save him; maybe, possibly, Remdesivir can help (clinical trials of the drug were on at the hospital).'

How does one take such a decision, that could decide between life and death, in such overwhelming darkness? There are no pre-planned check lists, nor prepared questions to base the logic on. Or is there a false sense of pretence presented with having a choice? How do you prepare for something you will never, truly be prepared for?

After a flurry of calls and phone conferences with medical professionals in the afternoon, the decision was clear to Manasi: either move me to the hospital or leave me here, and wait for me to die. She went with her gut feeling. 'We are moving Rohan,' she declared, her voice tired but firm. Was the decision based on blind optimism on her part, or was it a leap of faith?

Decision made, there were two hurdles to overcome— my vitals could endanger my body, and the usually blue sky over Houston was overcast with chances of rain in the evening.

The sound of a chopper in a hospital setting can be ominous. Loud, whirring, their blades shiny and reflective can send shivers down one's spine. It is a combination of dread and urgency; which doesn't make for a good cocktail. Isn't it funny how the same chuff, chuff, chuff brings about joy and anticipation when one is at an airport, waiting to get on a chopper to go for a holiday in a remote Maldivian atoll?

The staff prepped for my move. I was shifted on a stretcher, very, very gently. The staff let out a consolidated breath once I was completely on it. A minute mistake could prove to be fatal. The worried, frowning faces were all around. Some squinted, some took deep breaths to calm their nerves. Moving a patient is an everyday affair but not in my severe condition.

After fifteen minutes of observation, once the staff was assured my vital signs were as normal as could be, the stretcher began to move towards the roof. The chopper awaited. The hospital is not a massive medical centre, yet, every minute of the journey to the helipad for the staff felt they were cheating death.

I didn't know at that time, but Manasi, in her state at home, was praying to Sai Baba during that short journey. Bhushan, sitting outside in his car, was mumbling prayers to the rain gods to not let the skies burst open. My in-laws and parents were similarly praying in India, chanting to send me blessings to ward off all evil, the time difference no bar.

Finally strapped inside the chopper, I was ready to be taken to the hospital. It began to lift off the ground, the whirring noise deafening to the staff still on the roof. The wind was blowing, instilling dread. I had been blessed by so many people that I loved. But, would that be enough to save me?

For Manasi, it was those eight minutes of hope that prodded her to take the decision. Eight minutes of hoping was better than never knowing.

**The medical centre Rohan was treated with ECMO will be referred to as 'the hospital' in the subsequent chapters.*

PART ONE

ROHAN'S STORY

The Sneeze

I am prone to accidents. I don't willingly go in search of mishaps but more often than not, find myself in situations that involve doctors, medical procedures, needles, bandages and bed rest. A hospital visit is an experience I've had many times during different stages of my life that I take them in my stride.

The first such incident I can remember occurred when I was eight years old. My grandmother was walking out of the kitchen holding a large aluminium pot of boiling water. I had seen it boiling on the stove from afar when I was playing outside the kitchen. I was running around, chasing something. I don't exactly recall the game but when you are eight, any game that involves physical exertion is taken up as a challenge.

'Can you run and catch the ball, Rohan?' my mother would call out at Shivaji Park, close to our central Mumbai home, trying to get me to not bother her in the evenings. I would sprint towards the ball thrown in the direction, running as fast as my legs would carry me, and throw it back to my mother. The whole process would start from scratch, again. Till I was so tired that I was ready to go to bed. It was her way of dealing with my eager energy levels, her way of tiring me so I could doze off to la-la land the moment my head hit the soft cotton pillow, surrounded by my cricketing heroes as they urged me to finish off the World Cup final in style. Sometimes I hit a crucial six far into the stands for India to lift the trophy; at other times, I bowled out the opposing team on the very last ball, thus bringing a nail-bitting final to an exciting climax.

On that particular day, my parents were at work and I was alone with my grandparents.

I remember going round and round the kitchen table with intense determination until I ran into my grandmother just as she crossed the kitchen threshold. Her legs buckled, the sudden impact unbalancing her centre of gravity. She cried out in pain but my screams drowned out her voice. All I remember is looking up to see the pot tilting towards me, the intensely hot water splashing out in copious amounts onto my body. Somehow, my face remained untouched by even a single droplet but my body was so severely burnt that the cotton shirt clung to my body, plastered against the burning skin.

My grandmother quickly tore the cloth off, peeling away the epidermis, as a result exposing the pink below. A big mistake.

I was rushed to the hospital. My parents, uncles, aunts—they all arrived in due course. My neck and chest were bandaged up tightly and after many, many hours, once the doctor had done all he could at that point, I was sent home. 'No running around, young man,' he said, his face stern. Actually, I could not have run around even if I tried. The pain was debilitating.

I recall being devastated about being away from my friends. The fourth grade is a tough time in any child's life and to be away from all the action—friends, cricket, everything that mattered to an eight-year-old—was devastating. When the bandages were changed at the hospital every week, the pain was excruciating. I was one of the few to have been selected for scholarship classes but that was no longer possible. When my healing was finally on track and I could go back to school, it was still painful; I cried more than I care to remember.

My previous hospital visit had occurred when I was just three years old. That was necessitated by a headlong collision with a sharp edge, resulting in a cut above the left eye. I was lucky my eye wasn't the part of the body that bore the brunt and stitches in the emergency room (ER) was all it took for me to be declared fit to go home.

Fast forward to my teenage years. My next 'routine' hospital visit came when I ran into a scooter parked in the building compound while fielding during an afternoon game of cricket. I was trying to catch a flying ball, no doubt to prove my abilities like Kapil Dev in the 1983 World Cup final, whose running catch to dismiss Viv Richards changed the course of the match. Unfortunately, I made a simple miscalculation. I thought I could avoid the scooter and go around, bending my momentum like a superhero, but I was dead wrong. A metal part pierced my knee, causing profuse bleeding. After a hospital visit for sutures, I was advised bed rest.

When I was in my twenties, I came home from University in the USA to spend a happy summer in Mumbai. I was studying for my Master's degree in engineering at Lamar University (Beaumont, Texas) and was excited to spend the summer months in the warm embrace of family, friends and the Indian heat I had so missed. A day or two into the vacation, grand plans for the holidays still buzzing in my head, I slipped in the bathroom. It was no ordinary slip, my friends. I hastily grabbed the bathroom sink in a frantic effort to stop the fall; the old, ceramic white sink was unable to bear the weight of my lanky-yet-strong 6'1" frame, and it shattered into pieces. I fell on my back on the shards, strewn about in haphazard fashion, like pompoms and placards discarded after a celebration. A sharp piece pierced my back.

My entire holiday was spent in bed, stitched up, unable to sit comfortably even for five minutes. During a check-up at the hospital, my father, who tries never to show much emotion, choked. I turned to him surprised.

He shook his head and turned away. '*Beta* (son), I am glad you can't see the wound,' my father said, haltingly. It was a three-centimetre-deep wound, sore and painful. The ceramic shard had missed my spinal cord by just an inch. I still get shivers thinking about the near-fatal miss. Maybe it was in the stars, maybe I was really lucky… better not to overthink.

All these accidents, all these hospital visits, all the needles and stitches I had to bear, did not prepare me for the turmoil that was about to enter my life. Little did I know how my everyday existence would turn upside down, my family's life change overnight. This time it was nothing as dangerous as boiling water, metallic obstacles to cricketing glory or shattering sinks. All it took was a sneeze.

⚬⚭⚬

'This guy behind me just f**king sneezed. a**hole. I have a really bad feeling about this.'
WhatsApp message to Manasi Gokhale,
5:36 pm CT

I had just boarded a flight to Houston from busy LaGuardia, New York. It was 13 March 2020. I am not superstitious but it did cross my mind that it was a Friday. Of course, I had no idea then that the whole world was going to encounter the worst luck of the century. The number thirteen has long been associated with bad luck, a harbinger of evil. If the hockey mask-wearing, murder-raging Jason from the slasher films has taught me anything, it is to avoid anything that can go wrong on a Friday that happens to be the thirteenth. But there I was, boarding my flight to get home to Manasi and our three children, a routine trip I had done once every three weeks for the last three years.

I had taken up a lucrative tech job in Norfolk, Virginia, in 2017 but my family was still based in Houston. I was in a long-distance relationship—working in Virginia for three weeks and then spending seven to eight days in the loving arms of my family in Texas. I would take my kids outside, play soccer with seven-year-old Vivaan, go on date nights with Manasi, catch up with friends we had made over the last decade in Houston, spend time in Austin with my brother-in-law's family. You see, I had come to Texas to study in 2001 and never left, except for a brief six-month stint in New Jersey in 2005 for a job.

While growing up, I had visited the USA thrice, spanning the 1980s to the end of the 1990s. I recall having a gala time with my father's side of the family across the entire breadth of the vast country. I was mighty impressed by the lives my aunts and uncles had built in New York or California. As a visitor, I marvelled at how peaceful and independent their lifestyles were, oblivious of the hard work that remains invisible, brimming underneath the surface.

When I was on my own, I learnt how difficult things really can be. Balancing even a simple student lifestyle in a different environment with full-time studies is not as easy as films make them out to be. People say hard work makes a man but I say one grows up to be independent and hardworking when living away from the comforts of a family. That is when you realise how privileged you were. How lucky you were.

The world changed in 2001, America changed amid growing security concerns. From my aunts and uncles coming to receive us right at the gate when we visited the USA twice in the 1990s, to no receivers being allowed inside the airport, I have seen the transformation at close quarters.

Memories of an incident in 2002 still give me palpitations. I had taken a bus to New York from Pennsylvania with a friend. Marvelling at the phenomenon that is New York City, we began to take pictures like typical tourists with our point-and-shoot cameras. A policeman walked up to us, told us to stop, then escorted us to the police station. They took our identity cards to do a background check. We were eventually let go after an agonising hour with the cops. Looking back, I understand there were security concerns but the blatant disrespect and sense of humiliation still rankles.

At times the constant travel, the brief physical homecomings that ended faster than they began, seeing my family on video-calls without being physically close, the monetary stress; these factors all had the combined effect of making me dispirited. It was the first time since my marriage to Manasi that I was staying away from her for such long periods. The shift from the norm of my full-time job in Houston was tectonic. At the same time, I was torn: I am a workaholic who loves to do what I do. From the time I started my career after my Master's till my recent job, all has not been smooth sailing. In many companies for which I worked, the roles did not satisfy me. I knew I had much bigger potential than was being realised. There were jobs that did not reward me or even show me respect. I had to work doubly hard to prove myself. Whereas at Norfolk, working with my current company has been a reward for going through all those uncertain times in the past. I strive to do better every day because they have given me respect and trust.

Manasi and I talked of shifting altogether to Virginia, away from the southern city in which we built our life but that was put on hold for reasons which at that time seemed pragmatic. We would meet our challenges as they were thrown at us, we decided.

☙❧

The threat of the new virus overtaking the world was still pretty new in March 2020. In the USA, it felt like a distant threat. We had heard, of course, of the staggering deaths in Wuhan. The Centers for Disease Control and Prevention (CDC) tried to get their act together to combat this mysterious disease by starting screening of passengers at JFK (New York), San Francisco and Los Angeles international airports because these were gateways for people on flights from Wuhan into the USA.

This was on 20 January; the very next day the first case was confirmed in the country—a Washington resident who had returned from Wuhan on 15 January. Yet, no one was taking the matter seriously.

Before that, on 31 December 2019, the Wuhan Municipal Health Commission had reported a cluster of pneumonia-like cases. The situation quickly escalated, all in a matter of days.

Nine days later, the World Health Organisation (WHO) announced that pneumonia-like cases could have stemmed from a new coronavirus strain and issued a comprehensive package of technical guidance online with advice to all countries on how to detect, test and manage potential cases based on whatever information was available. The tone changed for the worse in the upcoming days: a Chinese doctor confirmed the virus could be transmitted person-to-person. By 23 January 2020, Wuhan province was shut down in an attempt to limit the spread; finally, on 31 January, WHO declared that coronavirus was a public health emergency. In just a month from end of December 2019, the world was reeling under growing panic with over 200 confirmed deaths and almost 10,000 cases of infection.

The USA declared a public health emergency due to the outbreak on 3 February 2020. The infection and death tolls continued to rise across the world, with the CDC informing citizens on 25 February that COVID-19 was spearheading a pandemic. The novel strain had met two of the three required specifications: sustained human-to-human spread and illness resulting in death. Worldwide spread, the third criterion, was still unmet. But that soon changed, almost in the blink of an eye.

The WHO director-general addressed a briefing in Geneva on Wednesday, 11 March 2020, two days before the weekend when I took a flight to Houston. The director-general was solemn. He declared COVID-19 was now a pandemic, and he was, 'deeply concerned by the alarming levels of spread and severity' of the virus. He also stated that WHO was noticing 'alarming levels of inaction' and that was what set off alarm bells. I realised the severity of the virus but truth be told, did not understand how terrible its effects could be.

Manasi insisted I wear a mask on both flights till I reached home, forty miles from the international airport in the southern part of Houston. I think she sensed how serious the situation in the country was getting. Manasi does not take things lightly despite her easy, outgoing personality. She's the yin to my yang; she's extroverted, I don't like to talk much; she takes determined decisions, I follow her lead. In the thirteen years (that number again) that we have been married, I have come to rely on her gut instinct. It's uncanny, really. She has premonitions and they always turn out to be true.

Manasi had FedEx-ed me a mask earlier in the week from Houston and I complied meekly, motivated by a desire not just to mollify her but also to assure myself that nothing untoward will happen. However, I still had a nagging feeling that all was not right with the world.

The fear was inexplicable, it hovered unrelentingly in Norfolk as I raced to finish an ongoing project for my team. It could have been triggered by a rumour at the office that someone in the building had contracted the virus on Thursday, 12 March. To hear this just a day after the virus was declared a pandemic does play tricks on your mind. A scramble had begun across the world.

The rumour turned out to be false a few days later but that day, the company took no chances and asked us to leave the building, complying with protocol. On the way back to my apartment, discussing the matter on the phone with Manasi, she suggested I fly back the very same day. However, my ticket was booked for Friday, the thirteenth day of the month. I sensed an urgency in Manasi's voice but chose to leave on the designated day. Maybe I should have heeded her advice, maybe I should have trusted her gut.

ೞ

'*Aabe koi* (expletive) *aabhi peeche* sneeze *kiya.*' (Someone sneezed behind)
> *WhatsApp message to Ranit Ghosh, 6:56 pm. ET*

I got a window seat on the Delta flight from LaGuardia to Houston. Initially, I was stoked to see the middle and aisle seats (18B and C) in my row empty. I heaved a sigh of relief. The earlier flight from Norfolk into New York was not crowded at all but once I entered LaGuardia to wait for my layover, I noticed how unusually crowded the airport was.

Ongoing research has told us animals can sense danger before humans. News accounts have published stories about thousands of ants fleeing the beach for forests days before the tsunami struck in Thailand, or elephants screaming and rushing to higher ground days before the waves destroyed coastal lives and livelihoods in 2005. But, like me, had other humans sensed impending doom that day and tried to move to a safe place before disaster struck? The airport was definitely more crowded than what I usually encountered during routine flights.

I was one of the very few wearing a covering to protect my nose and mouth. I was jittery, not even a cup of coffee could soothe my nerves. Instead, I chose to sit in a relatively empty corner near the boarding gate to finish some work—I needed to get my mind off seeing people milling about carelessly. I definitely was not in the mood to catch up on news from social media. If I had checked, I would have seen New York state confirm the highest number of cases in the country—421, with fifty of them battling for their lives in hospitals.

I didn't know then but President Donald Trump had, in an afternoon press briefing at the White House Rose Garden that day, declared COVID-19 a national emergency. It was the first time such a declaration had been issued in the country since the 2009 H1N1 influenza pandemic. The government said it would release funds, $50 billion in federal resources, to combat the virus and the respiratory disease it was causing that had already infected over 1,000 Americans and caused forty-eight deaths in the country. Worldwide, it had proven deadly to an exceedingly large number of people with over 137,000 confirmed cases and over 5,000 deaths.

'Through a very collective action and shared sacrifice, national determination, we will overcome the virus,' the President promised, as politicians do. However, he failed to take any responsibility for mis-steps that could have prevented the outbreak early on. There was also a promise of accelerated testing. 'We want to make sure that those who need a test can get it very safely, quickly and conveniently,' the President added. The Food and Drug Administration (FDA) had approved a new test from a diagnostic company that was supposed to make 'up to half a million additional tests…available early next week.'

As for me, I was just concerned about reaching my family. I wanted to go home and be with them before things got worse.

❦

I had barely settled into my window seat when I heard *the* sneeze behind me. It wasn't your average, nose-tickling '*Achoo*!', the delicate try-and-hold back sneeze until you can't anymore. This was explosive. An uncouth, raucous, hoarse sneeze that disrupted the quiet calm of the aeroplane cabin.

I almost cried out in annoyance. I was wearing a mask, I was trying to be safe. Why would someone else be so careless, especially when so many warning sirens had been sounded in the last two months? Coronavirus was raging in Italy with tolls jumping every twenty-four hours; Europe had become the epicentre of the virus, taking over the mantle from Wuhan; countries like Singapore and South Korea had already administered strict measures like aggressive testing. In the USA, schools were closing, Disney World and Universal Parks closed their gates, restaurants and eateries had begun to feel the pain of lower footfalls, phrases like 'self-quarantine' and 'isolation' were doing the rounds.

Maybe the passenger had taken Dr Anthony Fauci's recent *60 Minutes* interview to heart, where the leading expert and Director of the National Institute of Allergy and Infectious Diseases advised the general public not to wear face coverings because healthcare workers were facing a mask shortage and the extent of asymptomatic spread was still unknown.

To make matters worse, I could feel moisture droplets at the back of my neck. Being tall does have its disadvantages, I fear. My head always visibly sticks out and for the passenger behind me, his instantaneous discharge of droplets found its target with ease.

I knew right then things were not going to be alright. I texted Manasi, I texted my dear friend and colleague Ranit. I was scared. They say gut feelings are real. Why else would there be hundreds of films, in so many languages and from different regions, portraying the feeling as just and right? The protagonist goes with his sixth sense and ultimately, always emerges victorious.

'Stay away,' Ranit texted from Norfolk, enraged on my behalf. Manasi just told me to keep calm and come home. I really could not do anything at that point. We were on the runway, the flight about to take off. I could either worry for the next four hours, be terrified throughout the journey, or I could push out the negativity from my mind and steer my thoughts in other directions.

I may not be as expressive as Manasi and our families might want me to be but I believe myself to be a positive person. Soon my mind was flitting between Indian cricket, the project I had on my task list, the excitement of seeing my family in flesh, and the promise of playing soccer with Vivaan in the backyard. I cheerfully looked out into the night sky with its puffy silver clouds. I was going home. There was a smile on my face and a skip in my heartbeat, raging virus be damned.

Oh, how wrong I was. My life would never be the same, ever again.

That Awful Feeling

The wretched coughing had become incessant. Warm water, tea, even over-the-counter medicines were futile in combating its invasive nature.

The coughing simply refused to stop, having started a day earlier. Initially, there was an itch, an annoying irritant that was almost a tickle in my dry throat. In a matter of hours, I had intense spurts of dry cough. I went to sleep—at least tried to—but kept waking up because the nature of the coughing had changed to something more ominous.

The intensity was torturous; every cough left my stomach tightened, as if it was curdling my organs. My throat was so sore that no amount of water could ease the parched yet mucus-laden oesophagus. And to top this intense experience was the accompanying high fever that had begun three days ago. I have had seasonal flu and pneumonia before. But this time it felt different, even though I refused to let my mind wander to *that* dangerous possibility.

'It can't be anything else,' I told Manasi, firm in my own diagnosis, gulping down over-the-counter acetaminophens at the breakfast nook, keeping my distance from her. The date on the calendar stuck on the fridge door—held up by two magnets picked up from our travels in Florida back in 2011, a trip we hold so dear to our hearts—read Friday, 20 March 2020.

⳼

By the time I had reached home on Friday the thirteenth, it was close to midnight. My twins, Ayaan and Aria, were fast asleep, Vivaan opened his eyes for a brief moment before falling back into slumber. I smiled, kissed their foreheads and went to quickly grab a bite. The long haul on those travel days was tiresome but coming home to the family made every moment worthwhile. Manasi and I went to sleep talking about the mundane chores we had to complete the following week. 'Don't forget to call the plumber, Rohan. We really have to get the bathroom taps checked', Manasi reminded me just before sleep hit my exhausted body. I nodded against the pillow, mentally adding it to the list of chores and fell into the world of dreams.

I dreamt of the first time I met Manasi.

My first impression of my future wife was her determination—even before I met her. I had taken up a job in Houston after my Master's in 2004 and the next two years passed quickly. I was focused on my career, working day and night, not really thinking about anything else.

Like all Indian parents, when mine asked if I was open to finding a partner, I said yes. I was agreeable to an arranged marriage, so my parents began their search in earnest. They got in touch with several match-making bureaus in the country and began to talk with some families in Maharashtra. My correspondence began with some of the girls, whose details my parents sent me via email. Amidst all the correspondence, Manasi's emails stood out. It was not just her stunning photographs or her highly impressive educational background; she would make me laugh, she seemed to have a mind of her own, she was ambitious. Every time her email popped up in my inbox, it would bring a smile to my face, like Tom Hanks who would eagerly wait for Meg Ryan's messages in the movie You've Got Mail. But unlike Hanks who did not know who was at the other end, I knew exactly who Manasi was; I soon realised I was keen to meet her in person.

I flew to Mumbai in October 2006 and along with my parents, drove down to Pune to meet the Gokhale family. We stayed with an aunt who lived in the city.

The setting was typical: her parents, my parents in

the living room. Tea and snacks on the coffee table. The older generation discussed the weather and everything in between. Manasi and I carved out conversations amidst the overarching ones until her parents suggested we go out to a nearby coffee shop to talk in private. We were surprised because it was an unusual move in such a setting but we didn't question it.

We talked over cups of steaming coffee. Well, I listened mostly as she talked. I knew there was something between us. We spoke in detail about life in the USA, what it was like. 'Would you be okay staying in a new country?' I asked.

'My brother stays there, a large chunk of my family is dispersed across the USA, I definitely want to study further there,' Manasi said. She had mentioned that she had applied to a few universities, including the University of San Francisco. If she had not married me, she would have come to the USA regardless on a student visa.

Her determination impressed me greatly. She was sincere, proof of her hard-working attitude on display: there were no coy answers, no beating around the bush. As the evening turned to dusk, Manasi kept impressing me with every sentence she uttered, including her love for cricket. By the end of the day, I knew I would marry this girl.

'I don't want to meet anyone else,' I informed my parents the next morning. 'I'm meeting Manasi again later today.'

Vaishali restaurant on Fergusson College Road is

always busy. An attractive pit stop for Pune's bustling student community, the *dosa*s at this iconic eatery are a must-try. We managed to secure a table despite the breakfast crowd. 'I really like you,' I confessed, shyly, clutching holding on to a cup of coffee like I was holding on to dear life. I did not realise I was holding my breath until I saw Manasi's green-grey eyes light up and her face broaden into a smile. It felt a weight had been lifted off my shoulders.

I discovered Manasi's adventurous streak after breakfast, when she whizzed me to my aunt's place on her trusted Scooty, navigating Pune's jampacked roads with expertise, cursing at wayward traffic. I found the situation so hilarious that I laughed out loud, almost falling off the pillion seat. We broke the news to both sets of parents and decided to get engaged the very next day! I could not have predicted the decision to spend my life with someone would be so easy and at such lightning speed.

We got married on 29 January 2007 after a whirlwind, long-distance courtship. We stopped over in London for our honeymoon before reaching Houston. Her family is extremely close-knit and when she called them from a friend's flat in London, her tears tugged at my heart-strings. I knew I had to step up and be there for her, to make this momentous transition smooth.

The first few days of marriage were spent exploring the city and paying homage to cricket spots. I knew how much Manasi missed her parents.

⸙

'Do you think…' I gulped as I typed the words. '… it was the sneeze?' I messaged Manasi from the master bedroom.

I could no longer ignore the memory of the sneeze droplets that had spattered like Pollock's fervent brushstrokes on my exposed neck. A 180-degree turn from my morning prognosis.

It was afternoon and my condition had worsened. I kept popping acetaminophens for four days. It had been exactly a week since that godawful sneeze on my routine flight. I pushed away the thought of that irresponsible passenger completely, my days overrun with work, chores and family time since I returned.

I had just vomited in our master bathroom, and the thermometer indicated my temperature was now 101, over the century mark for the fourth day in a row.

I spoke to my father, a retired general practitioner in Mumbai the day my fever began. He suggested I go get some tests done. In fact, he kept insisting I go for a check-up but I can be stubborn when I want to be. I was in denial. I could not even fathom that COVID-19 could be a possibility but the world, in March 2020, was still trying to identify the symptoms an infected person shows. There were reports pouring in from news channels and social media, sometimes contradicting one another; there was fear-mongering because of the lack of scientific knowledge.

The very next day, a Wednesday, I went to the primary

care physician nearby and got tested for COVID-19, the flu and strep. The tests for flu and strep were negative but the results for the novel coronavirus strain took longer. No medicines were prescribed so I kept taking the acetaminophens. I emailed my company that afternoon, asking to take off on Thursday and Friday, hoping this flu would be over by Monday.

Rapid testing was barely available in the country, even after the President's announcement. The situation in Texas had taken a turn for the worse. The city of Austin had cancelled the highlight event South by SouthWest for the first time in its 34-year history; dozens of colleges and universities had announced an extension of spring break and the onset of online classes which had rattled the student population; the state governor had declared a state-wide emergency. Local papers and media houses were counting the number of confirmed cases but on 15 March, the first death in the state was recorded. A man in his nineties had died with symptoms consistent with coronavirus. Next day, Houston and Dallas city governments closed all gyms, restaurants, bars and clubs, limiting the food industry to only survive on take-out orders. On 19 March, the state governor finally issued an executive order through 3 April limiting the number of people at social gatherings to ten. There were 161 confirmed cases by the end of the day.

I dislike going to doctors. Perhaps due to all my previous hospital visits as a child, the threat of needles and injections, the presence of doctors, I have developed a phobia. There is a saying that unless one is at death's doorstep one does not take matters seriously. I thoroughly identify with the words. Manasi is exactly the opposite. She wants to go to a doctor for every little thing, especially when it concerns our children. 'Ayaan is coughing, we should get it checked', 'I think Aria is coming down with a cold, let's go to the child specialist.' I usually go along, reluctantly.

'Rohan, you *have* to go to the ER. You vomited, you have a raging fever, you are heaving and coughing. You need to get yourself checked,' Manasi shouted, her eyes narrowed. She was talking to me from the doorway. I tried to avoid her angry gaze, my head still hammering with a dull ache from the night before. After what seemed like eternity of a one-sided staring contest, I admitted defeat.

'Okay, I'll go now.'

☙❧

'What did you say? I have what now?'

I was too tired to be shocked but stunned I was.

I was standing with the doctor on duty at an ER close to where we lived. A decade ago, we had gone to the same unit after an accident and were pleased with their prompt service. So going back there to get myself checked was an obvious choice, bypassing the tens of other emergency cares services in the vicinity. (Yes, we live very close to many medical facilities in Houston, if you were wondering.)

The doctor had just run a few tests and informed that my body was experiencing an overdose of acetaminophens. I did not even know that was possible.

'The enzymes in your liver are high. How many acetaminophens were you popping in a day?' the doctor asked, slightly alarmed.

I had no answer because I really did not know. We, the adult human population, often self-medicate, thinking our body is experiencing nothing more than a common cold. That is what I was doing since the fever began and continued after my primary care physician did not prescribe any antibiotics.

I should have mentioned this earlier but from the time I began to sniffle, Manasi made it crystal clear that I was to go into quarantine in our bedroom. It was her sixth sense at work, once again. She knew something was off but could not pinpoint what was bothering her. I was bundled inside the master bedroom downstairs with enough blankets to keep an Arctic expeditioner warm, while she slept with the children upstairs in their rooms. It was a smart decision on Manasi's part to not expose the three under-tens to whatever I was experiencing. My chest x-rays were clear, I showed no signs of breathlessness but the doctor asked me to stop the acetaminophens and change over to a non-steroidal anti-inflammatory drug, available over-the-counter at all pharmacies. He felt the drug would help reduce the pain in my body by reducing the hormones causing the internal inflammation. In a fever-ridden state, I went to the pharmacy to pick up the drugs before going home.

On 21-22 March, I settled into a miserable pattern. I could not hug the children, nor play with them. I was locked in our room as they called to me from the other side of the door. 'Daddy, are you okay?' 'Why do you have fever, Daddy?' Physically, I could barely raise my head from the pillow but I would say I'm fine.

My symptoms were severe. I was constantly shivering, a new development that increased the distress I was already feeling from the incessant cough and raging fever. The anti-inflammatory drugs showed no signs of working their magic on my battered body. Every time I showed Manasi the mercury reading on the thermometer, as she stood near the door, I could see the serious expression on her face. I kept reiterating for my own benefit: 'Just the flu, Rohan. You'll get better tomorrow.' That entire weekend, my temperature ranged between 102.8 and 103.

I think Manasi told me that the Texas officials were considering issuing a shelter-in-place order. By the time I scrolled through news on my phone on Sunday, I was bombarded with the number of confirmed cases in Texas—over 350.

The world had changed in eight days, from the sneeze to my first ER visit. There was a growing hysteria in the outside world, like a Hollywood movie about an invasion by aliens: people knew something was happening around them, a fear psychosis spreading slowly but did not know the protocol for dealing with such a strange situation. Across the country, the situation was dire—the federal government spoke of expediting emergency relief funds as part of an economic stimulus package; California had issued a stay-at-home order, the first state to take the lead, and had also instructed the healthcare system to prioritise the sickest patients; the virus had been detected in all fifty states; New York was declared the epicentre of the virus outbreak in the USA with more than 15,000 people testing positive, making up over half the total number of infections.

In other parts of the world, the situation was grim—Italy's death toll had recently surpassed 4,000; in India, deaths were rising and Maharashtra, where both Manasi and my parents live, was overtaking all other states as the most infected. India had also banned entry of foreign nationals and cancelled all visas. When I spoke with my parents, coughing between every sentence, we could not believe what was happening worldwide. '*Beta*, take care, okay? You'll be fine,' my father reassured me.

'There's a Janta (public) Curfew in India,' Manasi exclaimed on Sunday morning. It was a voluntary lockdown in the country for fourteen hours. 'Aai (my mother-in-law) messaged me about the situation back home. She was asking about you, too. I told her your fever was persisting.' I could see her standing by the master bedroom door from the corner of my eye, as I was unable to lift my head.

Worse was to follow on Monday, 23 March. My high fever was stagnant, the cough was my constant companion, the shivering had increased and I felt colder than an expeditioner at the East Antarctic Plateau, coldest place on the planet, where a temperature of minus 128 has been recorded. I went to the ER again that morning. Full of despair, yet hopeful that they would be able to have answers on my second visit in three days.

The diagnosis was not pleasant to hear. My chest x-rays showed pneumonia. I was finally prescribed antibiotics to treat the symptoms. I recall driving to the pharmacy to get the medication on my way home but my body was refusing to cooperate. My brain was foggy, I had a piercing headache, there were aches and pains in parts of my body I did not know existed. I collapsed on the bed on my return.

☙❧

'You have to call for an ambulance if Rohan experiences any shortness of breath.'

This was my uncle's warning. My wife called my father's cousin, Milind Kaka (uncle) in Philadelphia, a medical professional with four decades of practice under his belt, to ask for advice that evening. He saw my condition over a videocall and despite my weakness, I could see his forehead scrunch, concern filling his eyes.

'Keep observing Rohan. This night will be crucial to his well-being,' he told Manasi, and then added: 'Are you okay, Manasi? You don't look that well either.'

I took a hard look at Manasi after that sentence was uttered. She was not looking like herself, I observed. Her face was flushed, her eyes were wide, and she was wearing a thick tee, one of those she reserved for winter. I think she was coming down with fever too and that was a kick in my gut. I hoped I had not passed on my illness to her.

I called my brother-in-law after that. Bhushan had come to the USA to do his Master's in engineering in 1999 and like me, had stayed on. He was in the north-western state of Idaho for over a decade and had moved south, to Texas, in 2010. He and Manasi are as close as siblings can be. He was a major reason why Manasi was eager to move to the USA, to be closer to her older brother. I have always admired that bond; in fact, the first person we visited after Manasi moved to Houston back in 2007, was Bhushan. He may be Manasi's flesh and blood but his firm friendship means the world to me. I will never forget the warmth he exuded as he welcomed me to his family after the wedding.

'I feel so helpless, man,' I vented. The situation was frustrating: Manasi was starting to feel unwell and the children were asking for attention; I was out of commission, unable to get out of bed to come to her aid. 'What can I do?' I cried, coughing as the words came out of my mouth.

Manasi gave the children their dinner and put them to bed upstairs. There were some tantrums, I could hear through the door but soon the silence of the night overtook the house. The three were sleeping soundly. Manasi parked herself on the living room sofa, heeding Milind Kaka's advice to keep a watch over me all night.

Despite the overwhelming physical evidence, I was still in denial about the severity of my condition.

ॐ

My cupped hands were spattered with blood.

This was not a rehearsed scene from *Macbeth* at the Globe Theatre but a very real scenario that had shaken my core. At 4 am on 24 March, I coughed up blood. I managed to push myself up against the headboard in the middle of the night because lying down was exacerbating the continuous coughs. My breath was laboured, my rib cage hurt with every inhale, my lungs were working overtime to provide my body with oxygen. The blood was the last straw. 'Manas…' I feebly called out.

Before I could finish, she was at the door. Her eyes were red and puffy, her face glistening with sweat from the fever slowly overtaking her petite frame. She could see my body hunched over, desperately gulping for air. I was delirious but still believed I could make it back to the ER at a more respectable hour in the morning. Manasi went with her gut feeling and dialled 911. She probably knew, deep down, I would be dead if I stuck to my guns.

The ambulance soon reached our doorstep, lights flashing, siren blaring, responding to Manasi's frantic call. I was afraid it would scare the children but I don't remember seeing them anywhere. The paramedics checked my blood oxygen level—it was 90 per cent.

Normalcy is 95-100 per cent; anything below 88 is a cause for concern. They came bearing a stretcher. I refused to be carried out. My legs were functional and I put them to use. I walked out slowly but surely to the waiting ambulance. The paramedics walked with me, ready to hold me up in case I fell.

I was taken to the same ER I had gone to earlier. This was my third visit in five days. Doctors immediately checked the blood oxygen level. From 90 per cent, it had dropped down to 86. That was not a good sign.

They needed to stabilise me before any medical help could be administered. I was given breakfast, I have no recollection of the food, but I recall taking some bites with difficulty. The doctors wanted to intubate me afterwards but my mind was so frail that I did not comprehend the severity of the situation. Manasi called me and despite my weak state, I remember her last words: 'Rohan, I love you. You will be fine.'

My fatigued body was telling me, 'Go to sleep for a few minutes'. I closed my eyes and sighed. Her words provided me with much-needed comfort in the medically charged environment where doctors and nurses were busy moving about, checking pulses, looking at test charts. Her positivity, the sweet tone of her voice dispersed all negative thoughts jostling in my mind.

I declared my love for her too. I thought I said it aloud but in reality, the words never left my mouth, I was so tired. As my body relapsed into sleep, to what I thought would be a short nap, I began to dream about

Manasi at the coffee shop. We were back in Pune, inside a bustling café, sitting across from each other with cups of steaming coffee between us.

And then, my mind fell into an abyss of pitch darkness; I lost consciousness.

PART TWO

MANASI'S STORY

The Scariest Day

I am a strong woman. I may be petite in frame, but when I roar, others better beware. Unlike Rohan, who is the most accident-prone person I have ever known, I am always in the middle of all the action and drama, trying to solve the problem and handling the situation. I think of myself as a seasoned veteran of many battles, I really do.

Once, back in Pune, my friend and I got lost in the bylanes of the city in search of a printing press for a school project. We had just stepped into our teens and with new-found freedom also came responsibilities. My friend started to panic, tense about being in an unknown area. I kept calm and kept asking strangers for directions till we found the destination in the back of beyond. I was not scared, I just did what I had to do. I was not trying to be daring but my parents praised me for my bravery when I told them about the incident.

However, the time I slapped a man for his inappropriate behaviour at Delhi's Jantar Mantar, my parents were taken aback, thinking of repercussions that could have followed. My logic was simple: How dare he think he can get away with no consequences when he groped me? It was a bright sunny day, I was observing the stunning astronomical instruments keenly, trying to soak in the history. That man ruined my moment and for that, I wish I had slapped him harder. I was not showing bravado, just being myself, handling a situation. Being a woman, you have to always be on guard.

My parents feared for my life in college when a creepy classmate began to send me letters written in blood. I guess he was trying to show he cared, but I was repulsed. Then began the deadly threats and the blank calls on the landline at odd hours. I felt I was being followed every time I stepped out. My parents feared an acid attack, a deadly weapon available over-the-counter at chemists. They pleaded with me not to go out, to stay home in the safety of the four walls. I refused to bow down to the terror tactics. 'How dare this stupid man play with my life?' I told my parents. 'I cannot stop going to college because of this. These are just empty threats because I refused his advances.' The stalking finally stopped; my parents were relieved but I was still angry that some creep could just scare my family with a click of his fingers. I wished I could have physically knocked him out cold.

Medical emergencies are not new to me. I have been through situations which no person would want to experience. I remember my father's first heart attack. He was always at the second-floor window to wave a hello when I came home from *kho-kho* (a traditional game) practice. But one day he was not. I knew something was amiss and climbing up the stairs, found my brother waiting for me on the landing. 'Papa is in hospital,' he said. We rushed to be with Aai (our mother) who was trembling as she sat outside the intensive care unit (ICU).

I kept calm when the doctor came to give us an update. I recall asking him what we could do to help our father. The initial seventy-two hours were critical yet, when I saw my father through the glass wall, lying on the white bed hooked up to machines, I felt no fear. I knew he would be fine.

Two years later, when I was fifteen, my father began to feel chest pain one afternoon. I was the only person home. I jumped into action. I called an auto, helped my father down the stairs slowly and rushed to the hospital. I handled the situation alone because I knew it could be fatal otherwise. I was later praised for my strong mentality.

I know I'm strong but in that moment when Rohan left our home in an ambulance, a feeling of utter helplessness, of dejection, overwhelmed my mind and body. I felt as if I had lost my bearings. I walked around the living room in circles trying to make sense of the crisis at hand.

I called Rohan at the ER to tell him I loved him. I could hear the discomfort in his voice, the laboured breathing. And that scared me but also put my mind at ease ever-so-slightly. I was relieved he was going to get treatment for whatever was ailing him but the thought of not being there for Rohan, physically, was scary. I could sense how much he was hurting; his fear of needles makes him hesitant to go for even his annual flu shot. I knew at the bottom of my heart that he was terrified of this monster that had taken over his body, and I wanted to be there with him, to reassure him that everything would be alright.

But I could not. Houston was closed, the threat and reality of COVID-19 having overtaken our lives.

☙❧

Rohan has always believed in my sixth sense. This intuition has guided me in the past, helped me navigate tricky slopes and it has also saved me. Call it premonition or a gut feeling, but every time my mind sends me a warning signal, my body suddenly tightens, my stomach knots up and I brace myself for bad news.

One such major incident occurred back in 1995. My mother and I had just dropped off Nani, my maternal grandmother, at her place after spending a lovely evening together at home filled with laughter and *pav bhaji* (a snack). We recounted many family stories. She pulled my leg. I recall we spoke about school and how the eighth grade was treating her favourite grandchild. I recall my mother in high spirits, her face beaming. Nani was sixty-one years old, strong as an ox, both mentally and physically. But I could not explain the feeling of dread that engulfed me as we bid her goodbye. I feared it would be the last time.

'Aai, I don't think you will see Nani again.' It was a simple statement, I still don't know what possessed me to say it.

My mother lost her temper. 'How dare you say something like that?' she shouted in the auto. 'Have we not taught you anything? You must never speak ill of anyone.' I had rarely seen my mother that angry so I kept quiet on the ride home, barely ten minutes away.

But my words soon came true. In two hours, my parents got a call saying Nani had suffered a heart attack. She was no more.

However, life is a sum of all parts. My sixth sense was a source of joy, not just sorrow.

Bhushan is my everything, the brother every sister asks for. Protective yet not overbearing, extremely supportive of any decision I take, ready to fight the world on my behalf if I'm wronged: he means the world to me. When he moved to Idaho to study, so far away from us in Pune, it was tough to be in constant contact.

When I tell my children about this, they cannot imagine how I grew up without instant technological gratification. 'Mom, you did not have a mobile?' Vivaan asked me once. He was five then, and I was explaining to him that Bhushan would communicate with us from the USA using calling cards. 'What's that?' was his incredulous response, as he played a game on the family iPad. He cannot comprehend life on this planet without technology!

As I mentioned, Bhushan's moving away was hard. Travelling the distance from India to the USA was expensive and the fortnightly calls were kept short. It cost a fortune on a student's pay. But in early December 2001, a year after we had gotten used to daily life in Pune without Bhushan's presence, I had a gut feeling. It was not the stomach clenching, fearful one. It was more positive; a feeling of happiness engulfed my body. I told no one, just kept it to myself. Sure enough, one fine morning, the doorbell rang. No one rings the doorbell at 5 am in a civilised society; it could only mean two things—death or disaster.

Our home in Pune is a three-storey building and my bedroom was on the top floor. Usually, I am scared of the dark but hearing the doorbell, I leapt out of bed and rushed downstairs. I ran into my parents at the landing, as they emerged from the bedroom looking worried.

'Who has come now?' my mother asked, her voice fearful.

'Why, it's Bhushan, obviously!'

'Don't be silly, Manasi. How can it be Bhushan?'

While I was trying to quell my mother's fearful thoughts of impending doom, the doorbell rang again.

"Uff, it's him,' I said impatiently, running down the

stairs. Of course, it was Bhushan, standing outside with a backpack and a travel-weary face. After all the excitement from the surprise visit died down, my mother turned to me as I spooned in mouthfuls of *pohe* (a breakfast or snack made with flattened rice).

'How did you know?'

'I just did. I felt it.'

Funnily enough, my instincts did not send me a message when I met Rohan. I was not looking to get married. It was not on my mind but after we met, my mother asked, 'If you say no, it's no. But what's stopping you from saying yes to him?'

She had this conversation with me the day we met his family at our place. Before our unexpected and interesting coffee date, I had exchanged emails with him numerous times and meeting him put a face to all the electronic conversations. Rohan seemed like a good guy. He was quiet, letting me do most of the talking; he fully supported my endeavour to study in the USA—there really was nothing on my part which I did not like. So, when my mother repeated the question, I did not have any answer as to why I should not say yes to the arranged marriage.

We were officially engaged in two days' time. Rohan went back to Houston and thus started our daily phone calls—my night, his morning. We discussed how to start our lives, clear doubts, to further get to know each other through our conversations. I knew he really liked me and I did like him. But I was not in love with him. Yet.

He laughed merrily when I told him how my work

at a governmental organisation in Pune was so hectic it would keep me busy till the week before our wedding ceremony in January. 'I didn't expect anything different, I know you love your work,' Rohan said. As I slowly packed up my life in Pune, Rohan made sure I was okay. He checked with me a number of times if my documents were in order to study in the USA, if I needed to get any paperwork done, boring legwork which will eventually prove fruitful.

We bonded over our mutual love of cricket. I had played during college. In fact, in the final of a major college cricket tournament, my parents were the loudest cheerers, much to my joy. I would never miss watching a match, nor would Rohan. His parents love tennis and had enrolled him in classes but he was keen on India's unofficial national sport. I mean, he lived so close to Shivaji Park where all cricketers practised, it was bound to make an impression on him. After he moved to the USA, he managed to play with friends there too.

Our mutual love for cricket was so strong that after we got married, instead of going to a normal, boring romantic restaurant on a date before leaving for our journey to Houston via London, we went to see the Ranji Trophy final where Mumbai beat Bengal by 132 runs (February 2007). It was such a pleasure to watch the likes of Tendulkar, Rohit Sharma, Ajit Agarkar, Zaheer Khan and Sourav Ganguly right in front of our eyes. I knew Rohan was excited to see Tendulkar score a century (he scored 105 in the first innings); he truly is a massive fan.

Over the years, whenever we watched matches on TV in Houston, just to get a humorous rise out of Rohan, I would tell him, '*Arre*, Tendulkar is going to get out on 99.' And that did happen more than once, no wonder Rohan thinks it's my sixth sense at work. 'Don't say that! It comes true,' he would respond.

છ૪

The medical team at the ER that Tuesday morning was finding it tough to stabilise Rohan after he passed out. They had intubated him but nothing seemed to work. I called Bhushan in despair, desperately needing to hear my brother's voice. This was the worst Tuesday one could ever imagine.

'They just can't stabilise him,' I cried, still overcoming the shock of the situation. The clock in the living room showed 10 am. Our children were up and about but I have no recollection as to what they were doing—whether I gave them breakfast or did anything for them that day.

Bhushan kept asking why. I had no answer because I had not been given any answer by the medical facility. Every time I called, I was told, "The patient is critical'. I myself had begun to feel unwell at the time we spoke to Milind Kaka. A slow fever had started to overcome my body and I felt weak. Ayaan came up to me some time in the morning and mentioned something about not feeling good. 'Mumma, I think Aria is also sick.'

I was constantly on the phone, calling everyone I

knew, asking them if they knew anyone in emergency care. I had to know what was going on with Rohan. Not knowing was driving me crazy, it was not helping my weak state. I was too scared to call anyone in Pune for help: Rohan was in ER, unstable; the twins were showing symptoms of low-grade fever; I was getting sicker by the hour—something was not right and my gut was telling me it was going to get worse. I just did not realise how devasting it was going to get.

It took hours to stabilise Rohan. When I found the reason behind it, I was furious. I called Bhushan, screaming, 'They found a leak. The f***ing ventilator tube had a leak. That is why it took them so long.' I don't swear often but the words just slipped out. I was livid.

Bhushan called up our medical friends and acquaintances, including our primary care physician. He repeatedly asked them, 'How can such a thing happen in ER? How can there suddenly be a leak in the tube? I don't understand.' He was scared, even though he refused to divulge the level of fear.

I called my mother in Pune after initially calming down in the wee hours. I laid down the facts—Rohan's fever was worse, his oxygen level was alarming, he had gone to ER. Every time I called, I was told he was critical. My mother tried to calm me down. 'Stay strong, everything will be fine.'

'I'm so scared of asking for help. What if it's not a simple fever?' My mother reiterated, 'You are fine. My grandkids are fine.'

Talking to her calmed me down slightly. 'Aai, please pray for Rohan. I don't know what else to do at this point.'

My family is not overtly religious but we do believe in the divine. My mother's beliefs are stronger than my father's and mine. She religiously goes to places of worship and consults with astrologers. My parents and I are so close that despite the extreme physical distance, they understand how I feel from my voice over the phone. That is why, I knew my mother felt my unease but did not want to burden my shoulders with her fears. I had, of course, discussed Rohan's fever and rapidly growing cough. They too, like Rohan, thought it was the common cold. But that morning, I could feel the fear creeping up inside them.

'Yes, *beta*. Of course, we are praying. Don't you worry about a thing, Manasi,' she said.

She later told me that in a little prayer nook near the dining room where there are many local idol representations and photos, they had put up a picture of Rohan too. They also lit a lamp to help the spirits guide Rohan to safety, which they did not blow out for months, until he was back home.

Bhushan had formed a family group on a messaging app to keep both sets of parents informed of Rohan's progress. When he told my in-laws of Rohan's state that morning, they were scared. 'When I got the call from Bhushan, I felt my heart sink. I felt a part of me just die,' my mother-in-law told me later. My father-in-law, scared as he was, kept shaking his head. 'Why did he have to be so stubborn? Why could Rohan not go to the doctor last week when I was nagging him?' he said on the call.

Both sets of parents wanted to jump on the next available flight and come to Houston. But it was not practical and not possible. India had announced a 21-day complete lockdown. The Prime Minister of India's announcement had taken the billion-plus citizens by surprise after the 24-hour Janta Curfew. It meant no citizen could step out of their dwellings except in urgent cases.

The same day, athletes gearing up for the mega-event of their lives, felt their dreams slip away—the Japanese government postponed the 2020 Tokyo Olympics till the summer of next year. This came after many countries had already refused to send a contingent to Tokyo given the public health risk and rising death tolls.

The world was a mess but all I cared about was getting Rohan the best possible treatment.

❧❦

The University of Minnesota had recently launched a clinical trial to investigate if hydroxychloroquine could prevent individuals exposed to the novel virus strain from becoming ill or reduce the severity of the infection. Getting Rohan closer to where he could avail the treatment was priority. In Houston, there was a leading healthcare facility in the western part of the city which had become a hub for COVID-infected patients.

Once Rohan was stabilised in ER, he was transferred by ambulance to the said hospital. It was already 5.30 in the evening and I did not know where the day had gone. I had not eaten anything, only drank fluids. My body had begun to ache; my children were cranky by the evening, unable to explain in words how the fever was affecting them. By then, Vivaan had also joined the sick bandwagon. Bhushan and Priya, my sister-in-law, were constantly on the phone with me. I had never felt so helpless in my life, the worry growing amongst us all as the minutes ticked by.

Once Rohan was shifted to the COVID Care hospital, I felt better. I thought he was finally going to get the treatment he needed to come home in a matter of days.

Why is real life never as simple as they show in the movies? In my favourite films, the director jumps through time to show the protagonist perfectly healthy in a matter of days despite getting into tremendous accidents or taking on an army of warriors single-handedly. The recovery period is miraculous, almost as if the protagonist had superpowers to just walk away with a few minor cuts and bruises when, in fact, the person should have been in the hospital for months getting treatment.

By that evening, I got the shivers and knew I was seriously ill. The three children were cranky, and to make matters worse, had begun to cough. Each time one finished coughing, the other one took over—a never-ending cycle. Rohan started getting hydroxychloroquine

Tuesday night but I was all alone with the children, unable to even step out. Bhushan could not physically do much from Austin, so he tried contacting friends whom we knew in the city. He was trying to organise someone to come to the doorstep to drop off some food for us. He contacted the Houston chapter of an international volunteer organisation.

Wednesday morning, a volunteer of the organisation named Madan Luthra stopped by with packed food for us. An amiable 75-year-old, he walked up to the front door, dropped the package, and then went back to his car in the driveway. He waited till I came out to pick up the food and waved. 'I am here. Tell me if you need anything,' he called out. Not just that day, Madan uncle was there for us every day going forward, eager to help us out with food and essentials.

My fever had touched the century mark. It was not the greatest start to the day. I was in mental agony, trying to chant a mantra my mother had sent by text to calm my nerves. Every time I called Rohan's hospital, I was informed he was still critical. He had been tested for COVID-19 but the results were not back yet. They tried to put him in a prone position—on his stomach—for about fifteen hours. The 'miracle' drug, which had shown effectiveness in some patients found in a study, was not really helping Rohan. By then, I had found out he was on 100 per cent ventilator support—and that had thrown me.

Standing by the kitchen sink, I drank two glasses of water to collect myself. I looked around the sunny kitchen and thought of my first days in Houston as the children called out to me from upstairs. My first visit to Rohan's bachelor-style one-bedroom apartment could be politely described as shock. It was not a romantic tryst where you are greeted by the love of your life after months apart. It was the sort where you could not believe what was in front of your eyes. There was one mattress and no comforter, two cheap plastic plates, a few spices jammed in a big plastic packet. I wanted to run away. I kept telling myself, 'Manasi, what have you done?' From being treated as a princess in a lovely home in Pune, I had come to live with a man I was still getting to know. Someone who was learning how to share a space with a woman.

There were depressing days, I won't lie. But after meeting Bhushan in Idaho soon after, I felt more relieved. My family is scattered in different parts of the country, including my grandmother in Denver. I would constantly speak with my loved ones during the day. Rohan's workplace was very close to the apartment and he would come home for lunch. I tried to keep my mind occupied by cooking Maharashtrian food, and in the evenings, go for drives around the city I was to call home. Getting used to the change was not easy but I had decided to move here, and I was going to stick by it.

Two months after moving to Houston, I got a job in the Indian consulate. I worked there for a year, swiftly changing departments, adding experience to my professional resume. I gained admission to a Master's programme at the University of San Francisco;

however, there were reasons I could not attend. I put my disappointment aside and did my studies in Houston, staying with Rohan as we built our lives. I did not want to take a loan for education, paying it off would be the death of me. I took up a morning job at a local newspaper which would help me pay for school and evening classes and gain valuable experience. I didn't know it then but the job would also help me make life-long friends. Rohan and I decided to expand our family after we were financially stable. First came Vivaan in May 2012, then the twins in July 2015. I was working in an administrative capacity in healthcare by then.

After quenching my thirst, I again called the hospital. There was no change. I sadly smiled at life—I was so scared to even order food at a Taco Bell when I first came but had become extremely assertive over time in the country I called home. I felt I could do anything; unfortunately, at this point, helping Rohan physically was out of my hands.

❦

Bhushan and I were in touch with Bindu Akkanti. My one-time neighbour, she is a doctor well-versed with USA's healthcare, internal medicine, critical care and pulmonary medicine. In one of our conversations, she brought up the topic of ECMO.

'What's that?' asked Bhushan. The extracorporeal membrane oxygenation machine is used during heart surgeries to help a patient's organs, taking over the work of the heart and lung so the organs can rest. Rohan needed ECMO because his oxygen levels were still low. He needed external help. Bhushan and I started inquiring in hospitals that had the machine without fully realising what it entails. I just felt in my gut that Rohan needed it, I was not going to question why. We asked the doctors treating Rohan on their opinion but their replies were not comforting. I felt they were not keen on making provision for it.

Rohan's kidneys started to fail the next day, 26 March. I got a call in the morning informing me of the situation. Bhushan drove down, not listening to my protests. 'What will you do? You can't come in.'

'I will be outside if you need anything.'

I had lost all sense of smell and taste and was suffering from nausea. I knew I had coronavirus even though no test had been done. Ayaan and I had severe symptoms. The USA, by the end of the day, had more confirmed cases than any other country—over 82,000 cases and deaths topping 1,000. Our family's news had spread in the neighbouring community. People were dropping off heaps of food, my neighbours called to inquire about our health, there were cards and flowers by the doorstep—it seemed we had the support of people we did not even know. I kept repeating I was fine, but I was not. I was delirious. My heart rate was high. Vivaan and Aria had high temperatures but were still actively playing around the house.

When I called the hospital in the afternoon, they still had not started dialysis. I was angry but could barely express my grievance given the current state of my fever-ridden body. The sight of Bhushan's car parked in the driveway brought me comfort. My heart felt lighter, it leapt with joy because my older brother was around.

Bhushan stayed in the driveway till late evening, planning to spend the night in the city with a friend. His stomach was slightly upset, maybe from the stress, so he stepped inside a pharmacy to get an over-the-counter medication. That decision changed his friend's mind. 'It is too risky to let you in, Bhushan, with the cases rising. You know how it is.'

While Bhushan was parked there, the news flashed warning alerts to stay indoors. New cases were being reported every hour, and it felt the world was caught in a death grip. Priya, though insisting Bhushan come to lend his sister support, was scared after the alert. Bhushan falls in the high-risk category. 'Drive home, do not stay at a hotel or go to anyone's house,' she said. So, after bidding me adieu from the car, Bhushan drove back another three hours and despite the exhaustion, sanitised first and put his discarded clothes in the washer.

I did not get any sleep that night. My fever was hovering at 101.3, my heart rate between 140 and 145. While Rohan's partial dialysis had completely deterred the doctors treating him to think of ECMO, a piercing call breaking the silence of the night shattered my thoughts. I was thinking of the number of times during fights I had told Rohan I did not want to be with him. In the heat of the moment, things are said that one does not mean.

At 2.45 am, I was informed the hospital needs to put in an arterial line to monitor his BP. It was coincidence or fate, but Rohan's heart rate that night was similar to mine. Was he trying to communicate with me through his soul?

In the morning, I could not get up from bed. My head was spinning, my body was hurting, my mind was lost. But I had to function, somehow. I do not know where I found the strength but with Madan uncle's help, I got the children ready to take them for COVID testing. Houston was a ghost city as we drove on the highways with Madan uncle leading the way in his car. The children were cranky and annoyed, I could not blame them. We waited for over three hours as Madan uncle tackled the excessive paperwork. The children had a scare when a lady in a hazmat suit approached our car with nasal swabs. The scenario terrified Aria, who jumped into the trunk of the SUV. I don't remember how I coaxed her to come out, the memory is a blur. I don't remember the drive back. I just recollect my hands shaking as I desperately clung onto the steering wheel.

⚬⚬

Life throws many uncertainties at you. But what we, as a family went through on Saturday, 28 March, was easily the scariest. I have no shame in admitting that I was terrified. I had never been in such a vulnerable situation.

Madan uncle had dropped off the doses of hydroxychloroquine prescribed for me and I had begun taking the pills. I felt my soul leave my body, I was floating in air like a bird, cutting through wind and looking down at the world. So small, so inconsequential. My phone rang, and my disoriented body, at first, did not know what was ringing.

It was the hospital. One of the doctors was video-calling me. 'The patient is deteriorating. Everything is going in the opposite direction,' he said. He was kind enough to show me a glimpse of Rohan lying in bed. I cried out.

His private parts were covered with a gauze pad and his declining vitals were displayed on the monitor. 'Any time we touch him, his vitals skyrocket. Administering CPR would not be recommended,' the doctor added.

I was firm. 'You will administer CPR as many times as required.' And then, I fainted.

I don't know how long I was out until Ayaan nudged me awake. 'Why are you lying there, Mom?' I splashed water on my face and called out to Vivaan. I sat him down and did the unthinkable—prepared the seven-year-old for an emergency procedure if anything happened to me.

I wrote down important numbers on post-its and stuck them all over the house. I unlocked my phone and explained to him, 'Vivi, if at any time mom does not wake up, you will take this phone and dial this number (911 on my emergency dial).' Short of breath, I was gulping for air as I continued, 'The doors are unlocked if ambulance people need to come, okay? Show me what you will do if I don't wake up.' I probably traumatised the child, getting him to repeat the steps over and over again. But it was a necessary step and I knew he would rise to the occasion if required.

I then called Bhushan in panic. I could hear the fear in his voice. 'I am coming right now.' He called up Rohan's friend, begging him to come outside my door to check up on us as he drove down the highway. The friend refused. 'It's too risky.' In frustration, he dialled Madan Uncle. Little did he know that the septuagenarian was outside my house. 'I can see movement inside, Bhushan. Be rest assured I am here till you arrive,' was his kind reply.

I began calling everyone I knew with a medical connection. My former newspaper boss, Krishna, knew of a doctor-friend who could help. Krishna was a mentor and close family friend. Over the years, he has seen my transformation—from a meek young woman in a new country who was afraid to speak up, to being back to my confident self, ready to go to the ends of the earth for what's right. He has always been a constant source of encouragement and is always ready to offer assistance.

Krishna called the doctor-friend in question, a much-feted professor and former chief of pulmonary critical care at Houston's top medical centre with over fifty years of experience. It just so happened that the specialist taking care of Rohan had been trained by the same doctor some years back. After he apprised her of the situation—a combination where a patient required dialysis and ventilator, both ominous from a prognostic point of view—the doctor began to make calls. Her call to the chief of critical care at the hospital helped immensely; they were ready to accept Rohan for ECMO treatment.

'I can send the chopper,' the doctor said, calling me back, and informing me of the huge risk factor. A patient on such high settings as Rohan's is not easy to transfer. First disconnect the monitors; reconnect to a portable ventilator, heart monitor, pressure monitor; then move the patient onto a stretcher and then to a helicopter or ambulance; issues, if at all, during the transportation; and finally reversing all the steps is an everyday occurrence in medical facilities. Even if utmost care is taken, there is risk at every step.

The medical staff treating Rohan were not pleased. 'It is a huge mistake. ECMO will not save your husband,' they emphasised.

I kept second guessing the situation. I prayed in front of Sai Baba's corner in our home, called my mother to get her take. '*Beta*, what does your gut feeling tell you?' she asked me.

My gut feeling was that for Rohan to have a fighting chance, he would need to be moved. The flight duration was only eight minutes but it was the only hope I had left to save the husband whom I had fallen in love with over the years. Leaving him at a medical facility which seemed ill-equipped to handle his care would be akin to leaving him for dead. And in the few days he had been gone, I knew I could not live without him.

I suddenly remembered the words of a neighbour back in Pune who read horoscopes and predicted the future. She had warned me never to utter words I would regret, to think long and hard in choosing phrases, even in an argument. 'There is something in you, Manasi. Your sixth sense or something, which can be fateful.'

I had fought with Rohan when he was in Norfolk, urging him to come home early after his office shut down. 'I do not want you to come home and then fall ill. If you end up quarantining, I do not want to be the one taking care of you, Rohan,' I had uttered in haste, angry he was not heeding my advice.

My words did prove to be fateful. I just did not realise the extent. And it was my responsibility to bring him home.

When It Rains, It Pours

My head was hurting, my body was fatigued, but I could not stop smiling. Rohan, finally, had a fighting chance. I closed my eyes for two seconds to say a little prayer, drowning out the noise the children were making upstairs. It was Sunday night and after days of uncertainty, 29 March felt like a little win.

When Bindu had called him the 'sickest person in Houston' the previous day during one of the group phone calls, she had meant each word. It was not in her nature to sugarcoat bad news but she would always end with a positive message. 'Manasi, hang in there. Nothing can break an Indian woman,' she would always say. Bhushan, as an older brother, tried to soften the negativity of the situation but I stopped him.

'It's okay, I need to know the harsh truth.'

I appreciated the honesty. We were drowning in pessimism and I needed to clear my head to take a decision. A decision that would change our family forever. I followed my gut. A quick call to Milind Kaka had emphasised that feeling: 'Manasi, there is no other option. You see a slim chance, just jump on it.'

Rohan's eight-minute chopper journey had gone off without a hitch—his vitals did not skyrocket during the move; the sky gods favoured the journey and did not burst the looming rain clouds hanging over the city; he was safely admitted to his new hospital that had provisions to aid his survival. The gut gamble had paid off.

⋘⋙

My body-breaking fever had miraculously disappeared Sunday morning but the virus had left my inner shell drained and sweaty. I was so tired; it was draining to constantly wipe the sweat streaming down my face. I wish it had been happening naturally in some exotic sauna in the middle of Lapland; unfortunately, the setting was my living room, and the children were still coughing and feverish.

'The doctors are still observing Rohan,' I told Bhushan over the phone. 'They will let me know once they do the procedure to put him on ECMO.' He had driven back to Austin after Rohan was admitted last evening, not before Madan Uncle had dropped off some homemade *rajma-*

chawal (rice and beans) at the doorstop. The joint calls with Bindu and other medical professionals continued all morning and in between, I managed to snatch a few minutes of rest. Priya and her daughter Siya video-called the children to keep them distracted so the adults could converse.

I received a call from the hospital in the afternoon. I looked at my watch, the time read 2.40 pm. They had put Rohan in a prone position, his oxygen level was at 90 per cent and his BP was normal without any vasopressors. They would start dialysis soon. All good signs. I closed my eyes to thank the divine. The prayers were short-lived; in three hours, Rohan's vitals were fluctuating, the virus ravaging his organs. His lungs were no longer exchanging gas and his oxygen levels were low. ECMO was utterly urgent, life-saving in other words.

Bindu had briefed Bhushan and me about the procedure in detail over the past days: how the machine works, how the patient is monitored and what he feels during the process. 'It is the maximum life support a patient can get. I really hope he does not need it…' her voice had trailed off.

Looking at an ECMO machine can be daunting. It is connected to a patient through plastic tubes known as cannulas. The procedure to place the cannula in the patient's large veins and/or arteries is called cannulation and needs to take place either in the operating theatre or ICU. Once they are placed successfully in the desired area—neck/chest/groin/legs—the ECMO machine is connected. The primary function of this machine is to pump blood from the patient's body to an artificial lung that adds oxygen and removes carbon dioxide, replicating the patient's natural breathing mechanism. The oxygenated blood is then warmed to body temperature, filtered and returned to the body. An ECMO specialist usually adjusts and monitors the flow in tandem with the patient's requirements. The two most common ECMO types are veno-arterial (VA) and veno-venous (VV). The VV ECMO is usually connected to vein(s) near the heart and is used only to support a patient's lungs. The VA ECMO supports both heart and lungs.

The patient also has intravenous catheters connected to tubes for administering medication and a breathing tube (endotracheal) through the nose or mouth, attached to a ventilator. The patient usually does not feel anything when first attached to the machine because of sedation. The science is life-saving but at first glance, the sight is supremely frightening for non-medical personnel.

Rohan's surgery took place at 6 pm. I tried to stay calm throughout the process but it was utterly nerve-wracking; Bhushan and Priya waited for my call. They had called our parents and Rohan's so the family could pray together for a successful surgery.

I was cold as I sat and waited. The mobile reception in our house is terrible so all my calls were being done from the washroom on the first floor, the only place I could catch decent connectivity. The master bedroom was completely shut since Rohan's departure and with it all my clothes and essentials. I was too scared in my current state to even enter the room; I had no idea what awaited me. The children were busy arguing amongst themselves, not bothering me with questions. I felt for them—their world had turned upside down. First, Daddy was ill; then he was gone and not there to comfort them during their sickness; Mummy giving instructions on how to call 911 and herself so tired all the time; constant phone calls; terror-stricken voices—had I been in their place, I would have justifiably had a meltdown. But they held themselves together, the band of three mini-warriors I was so proud of.

The phone rang. Rohan's surgery was done and the ECMO machine attached, they said. The large cannula was first placed in the leg vein and another in the neck vein to remove blood. The doctors chose a modified standard approach with two cannulas because they were operating by the bedside. However, it was a last-minute decision to give him VA-VV ECMO instead of just lung support. They had first attempted only VV ECMO for some seconds, but Rohan's body showed signs of hypoxia, a condition that deprives the body of adequate oxygen supply or a particular region at the tissue level. My heart sank when I heard that. Doctors then added another cannula in the artery to provide full hemodynamic support. They hoped Rohan would recover some function over the next few days.

Currently, with both organs—his heart and lungs—on support, Rohan was receiving the maximum possible care. Bindu's words came back to mind, echoing in a bottomless dark pit. But I was relieved as well. My heart was having an internal battle—yes, he was on life support and still critical but on the positive side, he was going to get better because of the machine. He had a fighting chance. Finally, the positive thoughts won, and the cold that had engulfed my body dissipated. I sat down with a thud, exhausted, but I couldn't stop smiling. I clenched the phone tightly to celebrate. (In two days, he would be transitioned to just VV ECMO.)

ॐ

'Next, we prepare for a plasma drive.'

Bindu's sentence took us by surprise on Sunday night. We thought Rohan was out of the woods; we were discussing the positives amid the despair and desolation around us on a group call.

'But…Rohan has just gotten ECMO…' Bhushan was stumped.

'It's not enough.'

Over a decade ago, a compound made by a chemist group was used to fight various viruses in lab experiments. A descendant of that molecule, Remdesivir, had suddenly come into the spotlight with the world in the throes of a pandemic. As scientists, companies and governments around the world had already begun a race to find a vaccine, clinical trials using Remdesivir had started at breakneck speed to see if the drug could reduce the intensity of the virus and ease an exponentially rising burden on public healthcare systems. The hospital was participating in one such clinical trial.

I had fought with doctors at the COVID hub who were claiming ECMO would be of no help to Rohan at the hospital. If anything could aid his recovery, it would be the Remdesivir clinical trial.

Bindu explained that because of Rohan's sudden renal failure two days ago and the need for partial dialysis, it was highly unlikely that he would qualify for the Remdesivir clinical trial. He needed plasma. Bindu was right, as I found out later: Rohan did not qualify for the trials.

Since this COVID strain threatened to take over the world in the early part of the year, there had been talk of infusing blood plasma from recovered infected patients to the sick as a source of treatment for the virus. Blood from recovered patients can be a rich source of antibodies. The part of the blood that consists of antibodies has been used in scientific research and treatment of infectious diseases for decades, from influenza to Ebola. It is commonly called convalescent plasma. Simply put, a survivor's blood plasma containing immune system agents aids the recipient in fighting the ravaging disease.

By end-March, the Food and Drug Administration (FDA) had finally given permission for plasma to be used experimentally on an emergency basis to treat COVID patients. Hospitals in New York quickly began to participate in such tests. An email sent out to Mount Sinai Hospital staff in New York, asking the recovered among them to consider donating plasma, drew over 2,000 responses. Researchers at Mount Sinai were among the first in the country to develop a test that could detect antibodies in recovered patients, which is obviously an essential part of the plasma treatment strategy.

The treatment was purely experimental at this stage. A reputed doctor and CEO of a New York hospital said in an interview with the *New York Times* that the key to the cure lay in finding the right volunteers—the donor would have to have tested negative and have no symptoms of the virus in their body for over fourteen days, plus have high levels of antibodies. The doctor said they would expect delays and shortages in testing because initially, the number of people who qualified would be low.

The process for eligible donors would be as simple as normal blood donation, albeit with a slight difference. The blood that is drawn is run through a machine to extract the plasma, after which the red and white blood cells are returned to the donor. The procedure is called Apheresis as the donor is set up with needles in both arms, one to draw blood and the other to return cells. Each 60 to 90-minute procedure can yield plasma to treat three patients. The plasma is then tested to check for infections or to see if it contains proteins that could set off immune reactions in the patient. If it passes the rigorous test, the plasma can either be used immediately or be frozen. When used, the sick patient would receive about a cup, to be dripped in like a blood transfusion.

'How should we go about a plasma drive?' I asked. It

was late and my body was ready to collapse. But I knew there was no way I could get any sleep; my mind would constantly hammer away at Rohan's predicament.

'Use your contacts, get all friends to ask around, call everyone you can think of. But a plasma drive is non-negotiable,' said Bindu, hanging up.

We wracked our brains. The end goal was to reach the maximum people in the shortest amount of time. Social media was honestly the best option but there had to be clear boundaries—prospective donors could not directly contact me: they would have to either get in touch with Bhushan or one of Rohan's friends who had offered to help. I was still recovering, I could not handle calls from unknown numbers and say the same things over and over again while looking after the children and everything hospital related.

We went to work at 11.30 pm. One of Bhushan's friends quickly made a poster for social media with our family picture. Looking at our happy faces, I smiled wistfully. Things do change in the blink of an eye. But I moved on from sentimentality. This was not the time: Now was the moment to be strong.

I wrote and rewrote a message to accompany the picture. I fumbled over words until I got them right with a little help from friends. With a click of a button, the plasma plea went live around midnight. I kept staring at it till my eyes drooped with fatigue. I dozed off with a prayer on my lips.

ॐ

Bhushan's phone first rang at 4 am. He was just hitting his deep cycle when the sound awoke him with a start. Usually a light sleeper, during this harrowing episode, he was barely getting any shut-eye. And the exhaustion showed on his face when we video-called.

'Hello,' he fumbled.

The call was from a concerned stranger, asking how he could help Rohan.

That was the first of many calls, the phone continuing to ring all day. It was a non-stop barrage from across the world, all asking a single question—'How can we help Rohan?' Bhushan sneaked in a call to me in-between rings, his eyes brimming with tears, stunned by all the sincere requests. He was sniffing, trying not to cry but I could make out the lump in his throat.

I went online to quickly check my post. The sun had not risen and the computer glowed in the darkness of the room. I rubbed my eyes at disbelief, staring at the screen. You constantly hear of things going viral on social media but you are never at the start of it. That role had reversed because in a matter of three hours, my post had gone viral with over 3,000+ shares on Facebook, the number increasing every minute. A close friend who had put up the post on Twitter found it shared over 8,000 times by the end of the day.

It was unbelievable. I have never been keenly active on social media, there is too much noise; when cyber space rallied behind us, I found my initial feeling to be one of shock. I was stunned by the genuine comments left on the post—comments reaching out to help us in our time of need. From family, of course, but also from thousands of strangers with whom I had no connection, just as concerned about my partner's well-being.

My eyes skimmed over my plea:

> *Dearest family, friends and well-wishers,*
> *It is my fervent prayer that you're all taking care of each other and protecting yourselves during these trying times. It is with despair and intense anxiety that I share the trauma that my family is undergoing right now. My beloved husband, Rohan, has been severely stricken with the dreaded COVID-19. He is desperately ill and has been hospitalised for the past week. His condition is dire. I want so much to have him return home to me and our three beautiful young children, all of who are under eight years of age.*
> *On behalf of my babies and me, I urgently request the support of the community in helping him make a full recovery. We are looking for a plasma donor with blood group A or AB. The donor cannot be currently actively infected (must have recovered).*
> *The ideal donor is someone who has recovered from COVID-19 infection in the last two weeks and is willing to donate plasma. We will be forever grateful! Please contact Bhushan at 208.xxx.xxxx OR Sxxxxxx at 832.xxx.xxxx if you are a possible candidate.*

It really took a long time for it to sink in that strangers were rallying for our family to be together, ready to help any which way.

Among the constant buzz, Bhushan received a call from a senior-citizen couple of Maryland who met the criteria. 'Just tell us yes, and we will fly down to Houston. We are only three hours away,' they said. A professor from Baton Rouge, Louisiana, said he could be a potential donor, having recovered from illness but needed to wait just two more days to meet the criteria. 'Don't worry, your brother-in-law will get through this. I am ready to drive down to Texas if need be.' A woman in San Antonio, one of the first to contract the virus in the state, said she would come to Houston to donate if it meant helping Rohan. An elderly lady from Seattle contacted us, assuring her support and her willingness to fly down, undeterred by the Texas state government decreeing a fourteen-day self-quarantine for any person flying or driving into the state.

Bhushan and Rohan's friend's phone did not stop buzzing all day. They even got calls from as far away as Australia and Singapore from potential donors who met the criteria. 'Can we mail you our plasma?' they asked.

Many messages on Facebook simply assured me that prayers were being said for our health. People were praying for Rohan in small groups, churches, cathedrals, mosques, temples and synagogues. People around Houston were offering to drop off food and essentials at my doorstep. Celebrities in Maharashtra retweeted my friend's tweet to their followers and my inbox was flooded with messages of hope:

> *'Hi Manasi, you do not know me. Some of my friends shared your post on Facebook and it moved me. Immensely. I hope and pray for Rohan's recovery and for your lives to return to normal.'*

> *'Manasi, my friend from Columbus Ohio wants to donate plasma for Rohan…Do not worry, Rohan will recover and be fine…god bless him.'*

> *'You don't know me, but I am Rohan's friend from India…we are all praying for his recovery. Be strong.'*

There was no ulterior motive, it was a selfless desire to help Rohan, and help us. Truth be told, the discovery that the post touched so many thousands was absolutely overwhelming.

Bhushan also kept getting calls from media organisations. 'Come to our show and tell us your story.' He refused, firmly telling them I was in no condition to talk to anyone. The local chapter of the international volunteer organisation Bhushan had first contacted offered instead to appeal on our behalf in the media. We agreed and their appeal helped draw attention to our cause, but it also soured the relationship that could have developed. They stated live on air that the children and I had tested positive when in reality, we were still awaiting our test results. That proved to be chaotic because in-between all the plasma queries, Bhushan's number was flooded with questions about us. The interview hindered when it could have helped.

Many local agencies had picked up the plasma story and published my plea along with a little background on their websites. In turn, it helped publicise the case when various Indian media outlets across the country reported the story. Rohan's name was suddenly all over India, with well-wishers calling both sets of parents to inquire about his condition.

The first post had a snowball effect. A snowball which first begins to roll down a hill is manageable. However, as it grows larger in size on the way down, it becomes faster and more powerful, sometimes unstoppable. That's what happened next; a misunderstanding that could have threatened my relationship with my dear brother.

⊂⊱⊰⊃

'The plasma drive is on. Great. Rohan will get what he needs. But what about all the medical expenses you will be stuck with in the near future?'

It was a genuine expression of concern from Krishna. I had called him to give an update on 31 March. Health insurance in the USA is costly. Navigating the world of healthcare can be tough, depending on the kind of insurance you have: private, social or dependent on the government. Apart from just medical expenses, insurance can also cover disability or long-term custodial care needs. The need for a sustainable and pocket-friendly healthcare system has always been a need but it still is not a reality. Child care, too, is expensive. A simple online search will tell you that give or take a bit, it takes about a quarter of a million dollars to raise one child from birth to adulthood.

Rohan and I have been fortunate in this mad world that is filled with inequality and injustice. We both worked to raise our three beautiful children. We had a house and two cars, food on the table and were able to indulge our children. When Rohan's Norfolk job came through, the constant back and forth was tough on all of us; moving the family north from sunny Houston was a plan we put off till our twins reached the age of five. We made lists, did pros and cons; it turned out, it would be less expensive to continue living apart than moving before the twins reached public school age. The plan was to put our Houston house on rent, move up north and put all three in public school together once the twins had passed the private Montessori stage. Of course, there was a certain amount of financial stress managing two households but then, that is life.

'You don't know the future, Manasi,' Krishna persisted. 'You don't know in what shape Rohan will come back. At this point, you can't predict the expenses. What if the amount is so high that you are left with nothing? You need to prepare financially. We must start a GoFundMe page for financial support.'

Everything he said made sense. It was true. I didn't know what the future held and could only hope for the best. It also played on my mind that I must be able to provide the facilities that Rohan needed. What if Rohan was unable to heal because we were drained of all our resources?'

I okayed the venture and Krishna went to work with an Indian non-profit he was part of, to create the financial aid campaign. Devi, the main coordinator of the non-profit, would later become a friend. She did not know us but continuously sent us food, with the help of volunteers, through the tough weeks, always accompanied by a personalised note to give us hope.

I managed to give Bhushan the update amid all the plasma-related calls he was receiving. He was also screening potential donors after getting more clarity from Bindu—the donor would have to be local; plasma could not be mailed; both test results—positive and negative—must be at hand for donors to be considered. I quickly updated my post to inform potential donors of these changes:

Latest update on Plasma Donor for Rohan Bavadekar:
There is no 'identified' donor at this point. The hospital system is working on protocols and approvals to make this happen.
Please keep looking for donors who meet the following criteria:

1. Based in Houston area

2. Must have been infected and recovered from COVID-19 with both positive and negative test results available

3. A or AB blood group (positive or negative).

I felt better by the afternoon but my body was still resisting a full recovery. There was no time to waste. I was gulping prescribed medication that had been dropped off by Madan Uncle a few days ago and making sure our plans for plasma was on track.

Krishna called to inform me about the financial campaign. 'We are ready. Just say the word and we go live.'

I stopped for a second to reconsider my decision. 'Would it help?' I questioned myself. The goal was to reach $100,000 (approximately Rs 74 lakh).

My gut said it would. Krishna was waiting on the line. I drew a deep breath and firmly said, 'Let's do it.'

✿

'*Arre*, how do you know this plasma treatment will work? This process is still being tested for COVID, nothing is proven.'

'You are harming Rohan. You should stop this plasma business.'

Bhushan was fielding all calls, answering the positive ones and being short with everything negative, all the while compiling a data chart of potential donors. He later told me, 'Manasi, there is no vaccine. If anything works for Rohan, plasma could be the best option. When there is nothing on the horizon, one has to keep faith in what one is doing. I knew, somewhere deep down, that this plasma treatment would help Rohan.'

Once the financial campaign went live, it got worse for him. On top of the plasma calls, he also had to deal with naysayers. And people can be ruthless when it comes to money.

'Why is Manasi doing a GoFundMe campaign? Do they not have money?'

'We have seen Rohan works in IT, Manasi works in healthcare. They have a house. Do they not have insurance or savings?'

'Bhushan, am I to believe Manasi and Rohan are so poor that they cannot afford any treatment? Is this a scam of some sort?'

'Is there some sort of hole in their insurance plan? We need to see the specifics before we donate.'

Bhushan was getting frustrated. He told one caller directly, 'Donating is not a compulsion. I cannot validate what you think you might need to be able to give money.' He told another, 'Don't give if you don't want to. It's a voluntary page, don't you agree?'

Bhushan acted like the big protective brother he is, shielding his little sister from all the negative rage that was embroiling our efforts. He did not tell me half the accusations these naysayers hurled at him. Since word of the finance campaign had gotten around back home too, both sets of parents were receiving calls about our financial condition as well. Forget the strangers and ill-wishers, he was having to defend the decision to create a financial safety net to our parents too.

Rohan was tested for COVID-19 on 1 April, and he had been taken off VA EMCO like originally planned. His vitals were stable and we had just gotten an okay from the hospital on using plasma for treatment. Bindu was a saint in managing the paperwork and keeping us in the loop.

It had been a little over two weeks since *the* sneeze, since our world turned topsy-turvy. I do not enjoy playing pranks, especially on a day which is considered Fools' Day, but for a brief moment I wanted to believe everything happening around was a huge elaborate setting for a trick. Someone would jump up from behind the living room couch and shout, 'April Fool!' like friends would in school.

I was still physically weak but on the mend. I could make out that recovery was on the cards. But there was too much happening around to find time to rest. Plasma drive and financial aid, calling doctors continuously to checking Rohan's progress, giving food to the children, keeping them occupied because they too were getting better. I would read out the warm messages I was receiving to make them feel happy, and give myself comfort. I know I am strong, I don't cry. But my mind was often straying to small incidents that, in hindsight, meant nothing. In the heat of the moment in a fight, there had been so many times I had declared I did not want to be with Rohan; the number of times I had gotten angry when he ate in front of the television set. Did any of it matter, really?

My phone rang and I saw it was Krishna. It had been about 24 hours since the campaign had gone live.

'Manasi, we have crossed the $100,000 mark.'

I was stunned.

In a mere twenty-four hours, sincere donations had poured in from around the world. Some names that popped up were known but the majority were strangers who had opened their hearts out of kindness and compassion. Each donation, whatever the amount, was followed by a message—they sent prayers, blessings and hope, they were all wishing Rohan a speedy recovery.

'We need to increase the amount to $200,000 (Rs 1.4 crore)'

Krishna would not take 'no' for an answer, emphasising over and over the heavy financial burden. 'You have three children, think of their future. What if Rohan never comes back?'

The asking amount was increased as I glanced at my initial plasma post. It had been shared over 6,000 times and counting. It could not be true, could it? The outpouring of love was overflowing and I, honestly, had to disable further comments because I was getting too many questions I did not have the time for.

ॐ

'We have raised over $200,000.'

I could not believe what Krishna was stating, that in two days we raised our target and more. He had caught me between hospital calls on Thursday afternoon, 2 April. 'We cannot stop now. We must increase the donation limit.'

I was probably going to say yes, but what happened next changed my mind.

I saw Bhushan was calling. Before I could utter a word, he began an angry tirade. I did not understand, initially. I made out bits and pieces before I calmed him down. 'Now, tell me clearly, what has happened?'

The agitation in his voice was clear. On a day that showed significantly high COVID-19 statistics in Texas and across the world, 4,660+ cases in the state and over one million diagnosed with the virus globally, Bhushan was angry. 'The focus has shifted from Rohan to this money business. It's not right.'

I was appalled. 'What are you saying?' I was somewhat aware of the negativity surrounding the GoFundMe campaign from certain people because a friend who was helping us out had sent me unfiltered messages but I did not understand the extent of the brunt Bhushan was facing. He was trying his best to get Rohan the plasma treatment but was constantly being hindered by calls related to the financial campaign. 'These calls are getting us all side-tracked. The focus should be Rohan. We can always campaign for money later.'

My quick temper flared up. I was enraged, my head spinning listening to the sanitised version of negative comments Bhushan had encountered.

'Send me the numbers of all the people who have messaged you such baseless claims about our financial situation; sent you horrible messages without even offering to help. I do not want their money. I will personally refund their donations.'

The arguments went back and forth till I decided I did not want to spoil my relationship with my brother. Siblings often argue, and we have had a lifetime of practice. But this one was different, I could sense undertones which made me scared. I had never heard him this angry. Quite unlike our fights on silly matters.

I called Krishna back. 'We need to stop.'

'No, we can't.'

'I don't want to hear anything more on this. I don't want all the negativity to affect Rohan. Please, let's continue this later.'

'Manasi, you have to be logical. You cannot let your heart be the deciding factor in this.'

I fought with Krishna till my voice was hoarse. I needed to sip on water because I was on the verge of blowing my head, metaphorically, of course, like angry cartoon characters. A puff of smoke seemed to be circling above my head.

As Rohan battled for life, I had become painfully aware that I could not live without him. But I also could not live without my sibling. And I did not want to do anything that could strain our close bond.

I made Krishna stop the campaign, refusing to listen

to his arguments. Even though what he said made sense, I just knew I would be lost without Bhushan by my side in our fight to keep Rohan alive. I kept my eyes peeled on the site till I saw the donation button virtually disabled. We had raised $204,004; much more than I could have ever imagined two days ago. Our closing message read:

> *May Rohan, our three children, and I offer our deepest heartfelt gratitude to you with folded hands and heads bowed low. 'Thank you' are words which fail to establish the magnitude of their sincerity but are all that we have to express the depth of our emotions at a time like this.*
>
> *It brings tears to my eyes every time to realise the goodwill that people have. Four thousand individuals, many unknown to our family until this terrible event—and many who decided to stay anonymous— stepped into action to attend to compassion's duties at a moment's notice. In the shortest of time, you raised $200k, an amount that we envisaged will scaffold the situation. Donations continue to pour in well after the goal has been reached.*
>
> *With the same sincere gratitude, we bring this initiative to a close. Thank you, once again.*
>
> *We are blessed to have you. You, in turn, are blessed to have the* daya *(mercy) that is within you, and the world, indeed, is a better place because of you. You truly are a strong foe, and a proven antidote, against COVID-19. We will eventually win.*

A few well-wishers have questioned, sometimes rudely, the need for raising such a large amount. As Rohan lies hospitalised in a continuing critical condition, and I try very hard to keep my three little ones occupied in the confines of the four walls of our home (for the past two weeks plus), self-quarantined and medicated due to testing positive, fielding medical questions and hospital staff, and balancing domestic duties while making immediate life changes, I'm afraid there's little need to address them.

Still, there are many things yet to be determined.

How long before Rohan is home?

What rehabilitation will he need?

Will I be able to keep my job?

How will all this affect our status?

And the kids...?

I am scared of the future.

I closed my eyes to pray for gratitude for all the love and messages we had received from strangers, who stood by us without even knowing us.

My phone rang, it was Bhushan. I breathed out long and hard, having come so close to losing him forever. 'Bhushan, listen...'

He cut me off before I could tell him about the closed campaign. 'We have a plasma donor for Rohan, everything will be alright!'

His words were music to my ears.

The Healer and
the Eye of Hope

My sense of foreboding was back. My stomach gurgled, warning of a coming calamity. I was snapping at the children for every little thing. I was on edge, just a push could toss me overboard. It was only 8 pm on 16 April but I just knew something was off. It was the feeling I had when I knew my grandmother had passed away.

It had been a tumultuous day, bringing a tsunami of emotions, but it was still not over. Bhushan had cried, my parents felt defeated, Rohan's folks felt all was lost. Everyone prayed: family, friends, colleagues, strangers. They all prayed for Rohan to heal, putting everything into faith. But I stayed tall, erect like a strong oak tree, not just for everyone else, but to keep myself sane. If I collapsed, everything around me would fall to pieces, like a house of flimsy cards. An early morning call had begun the devastation.

It's difficult to handle bad news when you are barely awake. My mobile rang at 3.45 am. It was the intensivist. My partner of thirteen years, the father of my children Rohan's heart rate had dramatically dropped while the nursing staff tried to turn him as usual, to save him from bed sores. Rohan's frail body failed to cope with the move. 'He needed urgent CPR' (cardiopulmonary resuscitation).

Just hearing the words brought nightmares. My mind flashed back to a year ago. I was standing by the side of a close friend who lay in a hospital bed, unconscious, seemingly dead. Medics were resuscitating him as best as they could. I held his hand and prayed. Thinking of my friend's bruised and battered body failing to come to life was heart-wrenching. I could hear his wife wailing outside, too scared to come into the room. It took the medics thirty-five tries to get my friend's heart pumping.

I could not imagine Rohan going through the same ordeal, the beating his chest must have taken with the constant compressions. I was fearful the compressions had hurt him more in his vulnerable state. I could imagine the torture he had to endure but I tried to stay strong though my heart was beating wildly. I could picture Rohan lying lifeless, and it brought back unpleasant memories, memories I wish would never reappear. As I tried to process the information, I did not realise I had cried out in shock. The caller tried to calm me down, his tone gentle-yet-urgent.

'We were able to revive him in two minutes. He is now stable. The cardiologist is on his way and we will keep you updated.'

I went down to the living room where Sai Baba's *arti* was playing. The sun was yet to rise. I sat on the recliner in complete darkness, the television light keeping me company and breathed deeply to soothe my nerves. Cardiac arrest and CPR were unexpected developments in the middle of all the overriding concerns but I knew Rohan would pull through.

❀

I had not stepped inside our master bedroom since the time Rohan began his quarantine. I would speak to him from the door, standing just outside. Since the fated ambulance ride took him away, I had shut the doors tightly and with it, all my belongings. I had literally been surviving on two pairs of jeans and three t-shirts which were luckily in the washer just before Rohan flew back. After I got sick, I did not have anything.

The outpouring of support for Rohan was immense, but it was the generosity of strangers, friends and Priya for the four of us that overwhelmed me. It took me a while to get my head around the fact that people are so keen to help. People couriered colouring books and activity-based toys for the trio; Priya, despite her busy job as a travel consultant, entertained the children every afternoon and helped with studies to give me a chance to rest; my best friend who lives in Germany called to keep the three occupied for an hour or so, giving me a chance to do my frantic hospital calls.

Priya, knowing my situation and what I could be lacking, did something which touched my heart: one fine morning a humongous package lay on the patio. When I cut open the packaging, the box revealed underwear, sanitary napkins, clothes, medicines and essentials she thought I would need. There were a hundred freshly made rotis packed in Ziploc neatly labelled with a note, 'When the kids are hungry, they can always have these with ghee and sugar.'

I had always wanted a sister, and when Bhushan married her, my prayers were answered. She may be my sister-in-law by definition but she's as close to me as my own flesh and blood. Much later, Priya mentioned that she was thinking of putting a monitor inside my home. Both she and Bhushan had seen me losing weight and my face going paler since the ordeal began. They wanted to be ready to help if I collapsed at any point.

Krishna, despite our previous argument regarding the fundraiser, dropped off food and snacks on our doorstep because I still had not stepped out; Madan Uncle would call twice a day to check on the grocery status and drop off essentials even when we had enough; my neighbourhood kept constant watch, day or night, over our house to prevent any untoward incident. I did not know until much later how much of a vigil they kept during that time, coordinating schedules amongst themselves. One day, during the first week of April, my friend from the neighbourhood dropped off freshly-baked cookies for the trio. It came as a god-sent because they could enjoy them with milk for dinner. It came on a day I was extremely frustrated with the hospital. Constantly hearing 'critical but stable' and 'cautiously optimistic' over and over again was getting on my nerves. I wanted to shout, scream at the top of my voice, 'Tell me something I don't know.'

Rohan's recovery seemed stable after we secured the much-required plasma, though fluid in his lungs was initially a matter of concern. Despite the fundraising negativity, I was also pleased that no cloud of pessimism hung over the treatment plan; the sole focus was now on bringing Rohan home, no matter what state he was in. I was mentally prepared for it; losing him forever was not an option. He received his first plasma treatment on 3 April. Bindu's updates from the hospital kept me sane—it was a lengthy process but once it was over, her encouraging messages kept the family's morale high. It was just the day after the blowout with Bhushan and I was on the mend. I was still hurting, mentally more than physically but repairing my relationship with my brother was the first priority.

The next day, miraculously, Rohan's vitals seemed to improve. He was still COVID positive, with the virus present in his body but all the inflammatory markers were better. We do not know whether it was plasma or something else but hoped he would soon be weaned off the ECMO machine. I was better, too. No fever, no shivers, no cold spells but the weakness remained. Among the three children, Ayaan's cough still persisted while the other two showed no symptoms of the virus. While Bhushan started to conduct more interviews for prospective plasma donors, I was trying to get Rohan's professional life on track—applying for short-term disability, speaking with his friends in Norfolk, trying to get a way to bring his Virginia life back to Houston. But first, I needed to figure out how to get his wallet, phone and anything he took with him during the ambulance ride. Everything was still lying in the clinic on the west side of town from where he had been transferred to the hospital.

౧౫౦

'*Beta*, the astrologers said Rohan will get better. It will just take time.' That was my mother over the phone from Pune.

Rohan's condition seemed stable to the outside world. His blood pressure was normal; a chest tube had been inserted once pneumothorax or a collapsed lung had been detected; his x-rays were better, he was given transfusions because of low blood cell count which we were informed was normal for ECMO patients; his lungs were stiff but that was expected in his condition; the ventilator setting was stuck at 40 per cent; his dialysis for renal failure was continuing; he had received a second round of plasma. As he had been transitioned to just VV (lung) ECMO, his current cannula configuration was one in the groin to remove blood and one in the neck vein to return blood.

We were in a limbo but it was a positive sign—nothing was deteriorating. Not even a frank discussion with the hospital's ECMO director could discourage me. It had shaken me, of course. I had baulked at the mention of 'end-of-life' protocol. ECMO was helping but it could not be the cure-all; what would happen if other organs start to fail? Usually, in these extreme cases, insurance covers two weeks of ECMO treatment. 'Doctor, let's discuss the possibilities if and when we ever get there,' I said, after listening to the no-frills, no grey zone talk. The bare facts were laid out before me in black and white.

My mother's call came at a time I was trying to get a grip on the situation. She mentioned, however, that the men who read the stars had given three different timelines for the healing process.

As mentioned earlier, I am not overtly religious but when my mother said she was consulting her bevy of astrologers, the only question I wanted her to ask was: 'Is Rohan going to live?'

My parents were praying all day. They would pray to all the different gods and goddesses they knew of and more, their altar was filled with divine photos and representations; their chants would keep them calm despite my father's blood pressure increasing during the tense weeks. Rohan's parents were equally worried.

Mumbai was under lockdown but they would find a way to evade local authorities to go and pray in the nearby Ganesh temple. The elephant god was helping them cope from so far away, when their only son was lying in hospital. They had put all their faith in the deity, risking the wrath of local police.

My mother's sister, Sudha, had put me in touch with a healer during this time. Sudha Mavashi (aunt) is an ardent practitioner of reiki and, in fact, surprised me when she said that she had been giving Rohan the alternative medicine energy treatment the moment she heard the news. She had had a dream early March.

'Manasi, the dream was terrifying. I knew something was going to happen to Rohan, that he was in a hospital bed surrounded by doctors.'

I don't know if I should believe in the premonition but was grateful for her healing energy. All the siblings of my parents, scattered across the world, were daily praying for Rohan's recovery.

The healer my aunt put me in touch with, Vasanti, had been based in the USA for a considerable number of years before returning to India. An extremely spiritual person and knowledgeable about the American healthcare system, Vasanti often felt something missing in her life. Until she discovered a particular healing method in a workshop in Nasik, Maharashtra.

'I found the missing link,' she told me once, during our constant back and forth of texts. The healing method was extremely simple: reading of affirmations along with holding a healing wand. Her healing was working for Rohan, I knew deep down. 'Manasi, I am not doing anything. It is the universal energy that does the healing through the wand.' This particular healing method was founded in 2008 by an engineer in Malaysia. All his life he had been on a quest to find simple healing ways to reduce the burden of the poor and improve their healthcare. With this healing wand, he had found his answer.

Personally, I believe in the powers of Sai Baba. I always have. The spiritual healer from Shirdi (Maharashtra) has been regarded as a saint among his devotees who are of all faiths. History does not tell us of Baba's religious inclinations but does it really matter? The man, all his life, stressed on the importance of surrendering to the divine, who in turn would lead the disciple through the maze of spirituality. Baba did not care for religion or caste, combining elements from Islam and the philosophy of Hinduism to impart knowledge to devotees. During the stressful week, I would often have the Shirdi *arti* playing in the background and various other mantras from YouTube. Like comforting white noise.

When I finally mustered up courage to open the master bedroom door, it had been closed for three weeks. I did not know what awaited me behind the closed doors. Was the virus still alive? Was everything still infected? Outside our panic bubble, New York had seen a surge of COVID-19 cases, setting a single-day record which was shocking and scary at the same time. A group of nurses in Texas were treated with hydroxychloroquine to see if they got better. The federal government had come out with the recommendation that people should wear 'non-medical cloth' face coverings, a reversal of previous guidance due to the lack of supply of masks for medical personnel. The epicentre, Wuhan, had opened up after a strict 76-day lockdown. India's death toll had passed the century mark. The world seemed to have gone crazy.

Wearing full body covering, rubber gloves, double surgical masks across my nose and mouth, blue plastic booties, a shower cap and eye goggles, I looked like a surgical ninja. No skin was exposed. It was late evening on 13 April. Earlier, during one of the regular hospital calls in the day, I had been told Rohan's catheter had been oozing so his heparin intake was halted for a bit. He received two units of blood and while his blood pressure was low in the morning, it had stabilised in some hours.

Bhushan and I had spoken with Bindu just after the hospital call. She had sincerely warned us that Rohan's ECMO treatment was reaching the two-week mark. 'The hospital might tell you to stop the treatment but you must push back. You must insist the machine be not turned off. Be firm.'

The bedroom was a mess– the duvet crumpled by the side, the pillows still bearing Rohan's head stain, his clothes strewn across the floor, bottles of medication by the bedside table. There was a lingering musty smell my masks could not evade. I looked around the room for a minute—it just seemed surreal. But I got to work, now was not the time to be nostalgic. I cleaned everything out, whatever could have possibly been exposed to infection. From Rohan's shirts to his socks, medicine bottles to the wastepaper basket waste, toothbrushes to bedsheets; by the end of an hour, I had seven large, full trash bags tightly secured. I slowly dragged each out to the garage to form a discarded pile.

The task had been exhausting. I put the children to bed and read them a story. I tried to keep my voice cheerful despite the heaviness in my heart. Then, I made myself a cup of tea, washed away the invisible grime from my body in hot water, and sat on the recliner downstairs. I was tired. And I burst into tears, sobbing like a baby, muffling my cries with a pillow, calling out to Sai Baba.

'Why don't you show yourself, Baba? I have asked you so many times to show yourself,' I sniffled. 'I need to know you are there, looking after us, looking after Rohan.'

I buried my head in the pillow, my body convulsively shaking. Suddenly, I felt something. A breeze, a noise, I don't know. I looked up, tears streaking down my face. And I saw him.

In the dark living room, lit only by the warmth of a single yellow lamp, there was a brief rainbow that sparkled in front of the television set. Then, Sai Baba's face slowly came into view in the middle of the rainbow and he smiled.

I blinked. What was happening? I could not believe it. Just as suddenly as the rainbow had appeared, it vanished without a trace. My heart stopped, my breathing became laboured. I had just witnessed a miracle. In all these years of my calling out to Baba to grant me *darshan*, he came to my aid when I needed him the most.

I wiped my wet face and straightened up. Somehow, deep in my heart, I knew things were going to get worse before everything got better. Baba was with me and I was ready to take on every challenge that was thrown at me.

❀

Rohan's cannula suddenly got dislodged. It was the tube connecting him to the monstrosity called ECMO. No one could figure out why or how as he continuously bled from his side. I got the call at 10 pm on 14 April.

Bhushan and I could not help but hear Bindu's words in our minds. Just yesterday she had mentioned a two-week period for ECMO and the next day Rohan's tube came out. Could it be just a coincidence?

'We have stopped the bleeding and put him back on the ventilator. The patient seems to have stabilised.'

'Are you putting him back on ECMO?'

'Not yet. The plan is to observe him and see if his lungs can handle functioning on their own. If required, only then will the doctors re-cannulate Rohan.'

I called every two hours, asking for updates. I was told Rohan was doing well but he required blood because of the sudden loss. I could do nothing more at that point.

My mind went back to the wonderful evening the children and I had enjoyed. For the first time in three weeks, I had stepped out of the confines of the four walls with them. The roads were eerily quiet, the highways as empty as a ghost town, as I drove towards the medical centre to collect Rohan's belongings. After days of pestering them, I finally got them to say yes, I could come. Houston was still closed. The shops were shuttered; restaurant lights flickered; the trio, so eager to be outside, plastered their faces against the windows for a closer look. But as I neared the ER, I could see their faces turn ashen in the rear-view mirror.

'Mommy, is Daddy in there?' Aria asked.

Krishna's house was nearby. After collecting the belongings in a trash bag, I drove to my old boss' place to say hello from afar. My mental health would improve to see another adult in real time. I was ready to stay in the car but Krishna came out, opened my car door and hugged me tight. His family followed suit. I froze for a second, unsure if I was giving them a death sentence.

'Manasi, if your friends are not there for you in your times of trial, what's the use?' He harboured no ill will about the GoFundMe debacle. I had the biggest smile plastered on my face as we all went to the backyard and chit-chatted over coffee as the trio ran wild. This particular memory will forever be etched in my mind. At a time when many were scared to come near our home, as if there was a mark on our door informing innocent visitors of the virus infecting us, here was Krishna and his family welcoming us with open arms.

That night I went to sleep still nervous but slightly content.

The shift nurse called at 4 am. It was a routine call, Rohan was doing alright. But I could not go back to sleep. My mind was still lingering on Bindu's words. 'What if they do not put him back on ECMO?' I kept asking myself.

The shift doctor who was looking after ECMO patients for that week called four hours later. I had drunk copious amounts of coffee to calm my nerves and chant the affirmations Vasanti had suggested. I had initially scoffed at what she said, how the healing method worked by connecting souls. But the more I spoke with her, the more I realised the healing powers of the method.

The way Vasanti offered healing was by imagining Rohan's soul standing in front of her. She would then request his soul to read certain affirmations she held up on cards, just for a few seconds, on his third eye chakra. These affirmations ranged from forgiveness (to help neutralise cords in health, success, emotions and prosperity), spiritual (increasing one's energy to connect to a higher self), to even one fighting the deadly virus. The entire process would barely take five minutes. The healing wand had a two-fold role, to heal and to sense. She would put my questions to the divine energy and the wand would either lighten or get heavy in her hand. Through all this, Vasanti was being guided by her mentor Avinash.

My faith in this divine energy was 100 per cent.

The doctor told me clearly that Rohan needs to be put back on ECMO. 'His x-rays are definitely better because I can finally see a part of his congested lungs but just the support of the ventilator is putting immense pressure on them.'

My next call with the cardiologist assured they would re-cannulate him. 'We will put one cannula through his neck.' They thought it would be stable. I had asked for the hospital chaplain to be present for any procedure done on Rohan. We needed all the prayers we could get for Rohan to get through this.

The next update at 4 pm was positive, putting all our minds at ease. The procedure went well; Rohan's heart rate was slightly high, at 130, but he would be under observation; the ventilator setting was the usual; there was no problem with oxygenation or pressure. Rohan was getting nutrition through his feeding tube.

But things never go according to plan, do they? The early morning call informing me of Rohan requiring CPR was nerve-wracking, to say the least. Afterwards, I got my bearings and called Bhushan.

'I'm going to drive down right now,' he stated. He knew I needed a hug from him but what was the point of driving down three hours when he would not be able to enter the house? I convinced him to stay put.

Word got around to the parents and I knew they were worried. My mother called her astrologers, my father sat in front of the gods, Rohan's parents rushed to the temple nearby. It was a stressful start but I knew after my recent Sai Baba *darshan* that things would be fine. It was a Thursday, Sai Baba's day. He would not let anything happen on this auspicious day. This firm belief kept me calm all morning while my near and dear ones fell apart. But I could hear my heart thumping against my chest despite my resolute stance.

Come 8 pm, an uneasy feeling of dread overtook me. I just knew something was wrong. I texted my mother, and then waited for the hospital to call. I completely ignored the texts constantly coming in from around the world. The children were keeping themselves busy, but I started snapping every time they came near me. Their disputes could wait. My phone rang an hour later and time stopped. My body turned cold after hearing the term 'CPR' once again.

The tube in Rohan's neck had come out during an ultrasound, shocking his system. It had happened around the same time I was feeling uneasy. With the doctors racing against time to put it back, Rohan's hemodynamics had worsened, and he had a cardiac arrest. Another cardiac arrest, two in a single day.

Twelve minutes. The doctors battled for twelve consecutive frightful minutes, forcing chest compressions until Rohan's body showed a teeny sign of life.

My heart sank, my body almost convulsed due to the shock. I could hear the children's voices in the background, as if far away but I felt rooted at one spot. I felt helpless, as if everything we had worked towards was slipping away. Every sign of improvement, every pointer towards weaning off from ECMO, all markers of good vitals—snatched away in a day. I still could not fathom Rohan's fatigued body battered twice in a 24-

hour span. I tried hard not to think of the high number of compressions he needed during those twelve minutes. Twelve minutes is not a long span of time. One can read a book chapter, finish a hot coffee, get some chores done, even a workout. But in Rohan's case, the minutes felt never-ending. I knew my uneasiness stemmed from something, but I never thought it would be this. I felt we had hit rock bottom.

I had to really, really try to look for something positive in all this. It was difficult, unbearable, but despite the backward slide, almost going back to the beginning, Rohan was back on full ECMO—the doctors had added arterial and venous cannulas.

Over the next few days, Rohan's condition did not show a miraculous improvement, unlike the previous week. The words 'critical but stable' seemed to be the only ones I was receiving from the hospital. My body was physically fatigued, my brain was fried. His lungs looked worse because of the chest compressions, which was to be expected. The doctors had noticed a large effusion around his heart, likely due to massive doses of anti-coagulation and inflammation due to COVID-19. The fluid was drained and his heart had begun pumping and was getting stronger. The high ECMO setting was also slowly decreasing which was a positive outcome. His haemoglobin level was pushing in the right direction.

Three days after the ordeal, Bhushan came to take the children to Austin. 'You need a break. You need to focus on your own well-being.'

They were fine, showing no major symptoms but I wanted to make sure they were safe for the journey and carried no harm. I had their antibodies tested and the results gave me relief. Bhushan came on Sunday, carrying freshly-made *pav bhaji* and *thalipeeth* (savoury flatbread). I could see in his eyes how much he wanted to hug me but I stopped him from coming in. I had packed their clothes in trash bags and sanitised them while wearing gloves and a mask. While the twins were eager to go, Vivaan held back. 'Mommy, you will be all alone.' I assured him with hugs I would be fine—only then would he leave.

I was relieved that the children were in Austin. A break from hearing medical terminology would do them good. I could use the time to pray and chant the affirmations, and just rest. After Bhushan's car pulled out of the driveway, I spoke with Rohan's cardiologist. Rohan's heart was pumping better, giving his doctors confidence that he was healing well, his body stabilising. 'We are planning on taking the current tube out and replacing it with a dual cannula for more stability.' It was a more specialised venous cannula from the neck that would bypass his heart and provide a more stable platform for oxygen delivery. In the future, it would aid in his recovery and rehabilitation.

However, there was a major hitch. Rohan was still COVID positive and the procedure was therefore not allowed in the operating theatre. That meant the surgery had to be done by his bedside.

I was flustered. Obviously, the plan seemed well

thought out, and I was on board. The surgery was scheduled for 3.30 pm on Monday, as the cardiologists attempted to get permission from administration and higher-ups. I kept myself busy that night listening to Priya's lowdown—the three had gone crazy in their backyard, running around and playing with their cousin Siya. After they had reached Austin, the three were marched off to shower and change before all that, though. And despite being tired, they were eagerly waiting to watch a Disney film, curled up with hot chocolate in the living room. I was pleased to hear that. I knew the past few weeks had been brutal for them, living in constant fear and unable to articulate their feelings.

The surgery was postponed to Tuesday for administrative reasons. I turned to Vasanti for support. 'Just breathe...relax and connect with Rohan's soul. Chant what I send you,' she said. She, in her own way, explained the emotional rollercoaster we were on, crossing one hurdle after the other. In the end, the ride would come to a halt and all would be well. That advice calmed my nerves. I would be lying if I said Rohan's impending surgery did not scare me. But the benefits outweighed the risks—there was a chance of faster recovery despite effects that could be harmful for a long-time ECMO patient. We had to grab the opportunity.

The next day started with prayers. Both sets of parents were chanting Vasanti's mantras, Bhushan and Priya too as their daughter kept my children busy. Krishna joined in as well as my mother's uncle, Ravi Mama. A Pranik

Healer had told me a few weeks earlier that he was focussing all his energy on Rohan from afar which greatly gave me comfort. I do not know if others were sending us prayers at that time, but I want to believe they were: it was a collective effort to ensure Rohan's procedure went well. The surgery was scheduled at 1 pm but when I called the hospital a little later, I was informed Rohan was still in his bed, hooked to machines. I desperately tried to call the cardiologist's office, but no one picked up. I was trying not to panic at this point. Finally, I received a message from one of his nurses at 2.16 pm: *'He just left for the cath lab'*.

'Nothing to worry about, Manasi. Stay positive,' I repeatedly told myself. I continued to chant mantras, eyes closed and breathing calmly until my phone buzzed twice at 6.38 pm. It was the same nurse.

'Just heard from Dr Sheth, he did well. The new cannula went in very easy; it just took a little while to stop the bleeding from the vein of the old cannula site. He should be back in the room from the cath lab in about 20 minutes.'

I heaved a sigh of relief and texted Bhushan to let the family know. Our prayers and healing techniques were a success, I strongly felt, with medical knowledge interjected by the professionals. When I finally spoke to his doctors, I was informed once Rohan was settled and off VA ECMO, the plan was to stop his paralytic dose. Dialysis would also stop and he would be given a diuretic to check his kidney function. And would you know it, his kidneys began to make some urine! Not even successfully potty training my three children had given me that much joy.

The reason for the shift in the surgery date, I learnt later, had a lot to do with literally building a plastic shield around the cath lab for safety. It had to be built overnight once his cardiologist got the permission to operate and it was not ready in time for the specified date. The humanity touched me. Not many hospitals or medical centres would do this for a patient. I may have been annoyed at the departure from the initial plan, but I had to be grateful because these medicine men were doing everything they could to bring Rohan back to me.

I desperately needed to see Rohan after the surgery. His heart rate was still high and his sedations had been stopped to see if he woke up in the next two days. However, another worry had crept in—did the lack of oxygen during those twelve crucial CPR minutes affect his brain function? A scan of his brain showed a bit of bleeding but was it a result of the CPR or an effect of long-term ECMO, no one was sure.

I turned to Vasanti, 'I don't want to jinx anything, but can you tell me if I should get a COVID-19 test done?'

My request for a physical visit to the hospital had been turned down but a FaceTime call was approved. I was going to be allowed to call on 24 April, the next day. I wanted some support by my side so Krishna was coming over, and I wanted to be sure that I was not going to infect him.

Vasanti's answer surprised me, 'You are negative. Don't worry.' And she was right. Before picking up Krishna, I went for my antibody test and was told everything was fine. I murmured a quick thanks to Sai Baba and went home in apprehension.

I had butterflies in my stomach. It was nervous anticipation, not dissimilar to the time I took my parents for a rollercoaster ride when they visited Houston in 2008. My father chickened out of a boat ride, drawing attention to his heart issues, but readily went for the topsy-turvy, death-defying ride. I was apprehensive about him but once the ride ended, it was Rohan whose face was white. 'Never ever again,' he had stated, fumbling to find his feet on the ground.

I chuckled at the memory. It had been over a month since I had seen my husband. I had no idea what to expect. I did not know what he would look like after all the trauma. I dialled the number at 1.42 pm and waited for the staff to pick up. The first look stunned me. Rohan's cheeks were gaunt, his eyes were shut, there were white tubes all over hiding his face. He was a poster picture for an illness that had overtaken the world, a virus that had no cure. I was all shook up but did not cry. I was sure Rohan's soul could see me on the call.

'I miss you terribly, Rohan. I love you. And I know I will be seeing you soon.' That was all I could muster before hanging up. And then I howled, pent-up frustration morphing into tears no dam could hold back. I was glad not to be alone, that Krishna was downstairs giving me silent strength. I was happy, of course, to see Rohan but terrified of what the virus had done to him.

'I cried, Bhushan. The man in the bed does not look like my Rohan,' I narrated in the evening. I could see the Austin couple holding back tears, understanding the trauma I was going through. 'But don't you worry about me. I will be stronger. I will not cry the next time.' Hearing those words, Bhushan and Priya broke down.

The next two days, I FaceTimed Rohan every afternoon. A COVID-19 test done once every three days, a quick jab for a nasal swab; his sedations were drastically reduced; tests were regularly done to check the level of toxicity in his body. I just prayed and put myself in Vasanti's hands. I chanted as per her instructions; I asked questions I needed answers to.

'Is there a brain injury?'

'No, Manasi.'

'Is he still positive?'

'He is not.'

My faith in her was rock solid but I was yet to get answers from the hospital.

Every day I called, I took a screenshot for comparison's sake. On 27 April, his cheeks seemed fuller and the tubes were still everywhere. However, Rohan had slightly opened an eye. I checked the time stamp. It was 4.13 pm.

He blinked.

I was over the moon. Hope washed all over me, making me believe we were on the right path. 'Don't worry, all is fine at home,' I tried to assure him, happiness spreading through every cell in my body.

Blink. Blink.

'I'll see you soon. I'll visit you soon,' I promised, sure that Rohan could understand me. It was painful to see him lying there helplessly hooked up to tubes but the joy of hope, the hope that he was finally conscious, was unmatchable. The cardiologist had warned me after the surgery that if and when Rohan woke up, no one would have any idea what shape he would be in, reiterating that he had never seen a patient as sick as my partner. At that moment, I did not care about the doctor's caution or anything for that matter. Everything we had worked towards over the last month had resulted in an open eye. We had worked our way up from the depths of the cold rocky bottom of two cardiac arrests. That was the hope I was clinging onto.

What made the day even sweeter was the result of Rohan's latest COVID-19 test. Hearing the word 'negative' for the first time brought fresh tears. For the first time in a long while, they were tears of happiness.

Promises to Keep

'When will Daddy come home?'

It was such an innocent question but it broke my heart to explain to the birthday boy that I simply had no idea.

Vivaan was celebrating his eighth birthday. A birthday is supposed to be fun, a day of frolic and mirth with friends, ice cream and intense running around the backyard. Unfortunately, 2020 was not the year for merriment. Rohan and I had discussed the three children's birthdays, and how we could celebrate over the summer last November. We had come home after spending three wonderful weeks in India, splitting our time between Mumbai and Pune. We had also performed Vivaan's *Upanayanam* there, a traditional thread ceremony which our families consider sacred. The children had had a blast meeting their grandparents. They were spoilt rotten, getting everything handed to them, no demand too great. It was during one such evening in Pune that my parents had brought up the topic of the trio's birthdays next summer.

'We are hoping to come in April and stay on till the twins' birthdays in July. We will definitely spend some time in Denver with your grandmother and aunt; and how about a weekend trip with the kids to a beach? Maybe, we could do a beach celebration for Vivi?'

Rohan and I had given my father's idea a lot of thought. 'I can take leave for a couple of days,' Rohan said. I, too, agreed. In our family text thread, we had put forth a couple of places we could have gone for a long weekend of celebrations.

I recalled my father's words on the morning of 1 May. It was a Friday. The eighth birthday that could have been.

⚭

After the regaining of joy three days ago, of relief combined with happiness that left me floating on cloud nine, the mood hit a snag. Rohan opening one eye was a good omen but he was not even near the edge of Amazonian-sized woods. There was a lot of work that needed to be done but the pace depended on his battered body.

The doctor on duty had pointed out that while his right eye had opened briefly, Rohan's left eye pupil was unreactive. They wanted to run more tests to see how his brain was coping after he awoke. The doctors had earlier suggested Rohan might have suffered a minor stroke. But they would only be able to pinpoint the location once he regained consciousness. Unfortunately, they found something alarming.

The location of the stroke was crucial—at the left back of his brain, the area responsible for cognitive functioning in a human. I would lie if I didn't say hearing the diagnosis was a bummer. Recovery was on track, the plasma treatment seemed to indicate positive signs of recovery which had even been reported by media outlets, the surgery went well, everything that could have gone wrong, did not. And now this.

I needed a hug. I called my mother just to talk, needing an outlet to vent my frustration. The whole journey seemed so topsy-turvy that I couldn't take anything for granted. I could hear her tired voice trying to calm me down. From the very beginning, they had not regarded Rohan as a son-in-law but a son. Despite his taciturn nature, they embraced him into their fold. And I knew how badly they must be hurting now, being so far away.

That night I spoke with the children who were still in Austin. They would ask me how Daddy was, interrupting either Bhushan or Priya in the middle of the call, every time I called with an update. They were too young, of course, but obviously could sense the urgency of the situation.

'Vivi, Daddy is better. I promise he will speak with you once he gets even better,' I reassured the eldest. To the twins: 'Daddy loves you very much. He will come home, soon.' I completely believed in the words I uttered. I was mentally prepared that Rohan would not be coming back at 100 per cent capacity but I was sure that he would be coming home some day.

Rohan's progress was even better the next day. He had opened both his eyes in the morning. The nurse on duty mentioned Rohan's mouth was showing signs of a grimace and he was feebly attempting to move his right arm.

When I FaceTimed him in the afternoon, Rohan's eyes were still droopy but they both opened, albeit briefly. I could feel some sense of relief at that moment. However, suddenly, he started gagging, choking on the tube in his mouth. My eyes went wide with fear and I began to shout out to the nurse, who was holding the phone, to help him. After soothing him down, the nurse turned the camera towards her face and I was completely taken aback by her smile.

'Ma'am, this is a wonderful sign!' She elaborated that Rohan gagging meant he was getting back sensations. He could feel the tubes. This, coupled with his arm movements, were all wins for us.

'Look, see this,' the nurse added. Turning to Rohan, she asked him to squeeze her hand. I could make out his reflex motion, though barely. He had heard her, and was trying to follow instructions! 'His brain is functioning,' I thought to myself. When I narrated the day's proceedings to Bhushan, I could see the joy creeping up on his face. 'This is it; we must keep fighting,' he said, eyes sparkling. I could hear the children happily playing in the background. 'They are busy outside drawing with chalk. I also played a little soccer with Vivi. I knew he was missing it,' he added.

Vivaan shares a love of sports with Rohan. Soccer, tennis, cricket, anything that involves running and chasing a ball. Previously, every afternoon that Rohan spent at Houston had the father-son duo kicking a ball in the backyard. Rohan had set up a tiny goalpost at one end, and I would see them trying to outdo one another in trying to score. Sometimes, they would completely forget the time and keep playing, which did annoy me. Still, that scenario was any day preferable to the hospital business.

Rohan's kidneys were functioning and he was producing at least 190 ml of urine. He was COVID-19 negative and there was talk of moving him to the normal ICU from the speciality coronavirus the next day. However, he was still on VV ECMO. I hoped against hope he would be off the machine in the next two days, in time for Vivaan's birthday.

On 30 April, the hospital called to say they wanted to perform a tracheostomy on Rohan. During my candid chat with the doctors earlier in the month, I had been explained the necessary steps to take if he came off the ECMO machine. Now that he had woken up, and his brain and kidneys were functioning, the next step was to get him to move his limbs. They wanted to do this temporary procedure because of his long-term dependency on a ventilator for lung function. The key function of performing this surgical procedure is simple—make a hole through the front of the neck and into a windpipe, and place a tube in it to aid breathing. It creates an air passage when the natural route for breathing is hampered. They would also put in a peg tube at the same time for feeding—killing two birds with one stone.

'We are taking baby steps in the right direction,' I was assured.

I called Vasanti. 'Is it necessary to do the procedure today?' she questioned.

The urgency in her voice surprised me. 'Why, Vasanti? Is something wrong with Rohan? Is it going to be a risk?'

'It is not a good day. Can you wait till tomorrow?'

When the hospital called me back and asked for permission, I could not refuse consent. I had no medical reason to hold off. No matter my firm beliefs, I could not tell them to put off the surgery based on a feeling or that the day was not right. It would make no sense.

I kept pacing up and down the living room, waiting with uncertainty. My gut feeling did not make an appearance on this occasion but the healer's words kept coming back. 'Did I do the right thing?' I asked myself over and over again. My father called in the middle of my agitation. His demeanour was different and after much coaxing, he revealed his blood pressure had shot up the last two days due to the anxiety and lack of sleep. His words were worrisome, especially when I heard my mother scold him over the phone, 'Stop worrying, Manasi.'

My phone rang at 3:30 pm. 'The tracheostomy was a success.'

It was a relief but I still couldn't get Vasanti's words out of my head. It didn't feel right.

The next call, that came in half an hour later, made my breathing laboured. 'We need your consent to take the patient to the OR (operating room). We have no time to waste.'

I sat still on the recliner and prayed. Some mantra was playing on my laptop in the background; the children called it 'Daddy's song' thinking the amalgamation of chants to be one. It was a Thursday, Sai Baba's day. After coming to see me, I knew he would not betray me on his holy day. But my anxiousness overrode my thinking. I breathed in and out slowly, trying to calm myself down. I realised my body was shivering slightly with dread. There was a sinking feeling at the pit of my stomach.

The call that came after an hour brought with it some relief. I learned that after the tubes were inserted into Rohan's trachea and the procedure was okayed, his blood pressure was still low. They gave him blood, up to five units, yet it did not stabilise him. So they rushed to the OR and cut open his stomach. In trying to put in the feeding peg tube, a capillary had broken, causing internal bleeding in his stomach. Finally, after a day of medically wrestling against the clock, Rohan's vitals were stabilised and he seemed fine.

I just shook my head after the hospital call and admonished myself, 'Why didn't you listen to Vasanti? Why?'

I strictly told Bhushan, when he came in the evening to drop off the trio, not to divulge the details of the sudden surgery to our parents. What if something happened to our father after hearing about the bleeding? Things were okay, and it was time to think of the future. There was no point worrying about 'what could have been'.

⳨

Rohan had been very close to his paternal grandfather. I remember the way he spoke about his 'Aaba' on our first 'coffee date'. Animated, expressive, his eyes had a sparkle; I could also sense he still carried the hurt of losing him. It was his Aaba who had inculcated in him his love for cricket, from taking him to practice at Shivaji Park to sharing his nuanced wisdom watching matches on the television set. Rohan would do anything his Aaba asked him to. He told me in detail about the gentle manner Aaba would hold the attention of anyone with whom he spoke.

His love for his family was probably one of the reasons that attracted me to his quiet nature. He always showed his love, he did not say much. I recall laughing hard while eating a takeout Chinese dinner sitting on the floor in our Houston apartment as he narrated a story about his grandfather.

Aaba had needed physical therapy for a lingering neck pain and Rohan would accompany him to the doctor every time. On one such visit, the discussion had turned to cricket, and Aaba had mentioned how the national cricket team needed new blood. 'I think Sanjay Manjrekar should be included.' Manjrekar was then a big name in the domestic circuit, yet to make his mark internationally. 'Oh, do you want to meet him? He is here at the clinic.' Rohan narrated how both he and Aaba had gotten excited at the chance of meeting a cricketer; Aaba more so, completely forgetting his neck pain, nodding vehemently—much to the doctor's surprise!

His mother later told me how Rohan had taken charge of looking after his Aaba when he was diagnosed with Alzheimer's. 'Rohan was just out of college when that happened. We arranged for nurses because his father and I both worked but that did not deter Rohan. He would ensure his grandfather was alright, bringing him medicines, spending every single free hour with him, just to make sure he got proper care. After he passed away, Rohan was crushed but because he barely spoke, he threw himself into studies and sports. Whatever he chose to do, he gave his 100 per cent, as his Aaba had taught him.'

We had decided to wait for some years to start a family, until we were financially stable with a double income. Our parents had come to the USA to help when Vivaan was born in 2012 and starting his first day on the planet, was spoilt by both sets of grandparents. For three years before the twins came, he was Rohan's entire world. Rohan tried to inculcate a sporting passion into Vivaan like his grandfather had done for him. It worked wonders. Since the time Vivaan could kick a ball, Rohan would be chasing him around, encouraging him to kick it as hard as he could. As he got older, Rohan would take him to the tennis courts near our house for lessons. He enjoyed practising the forehand but once he discovered Cristiano Ronaldo, there was no looking back. Just as Rohan would practice at Shivaji Park idolising Tendulkar, Vivi would spend hours at soccer practice, both at lessons and in the backyard, pushing himself like Ronaldo.

The memory of the day Rohan took him for his first local game in Houston brings a smile to my face. He was barely four and did not understand the rules or what exactly was happening but Rohan told me how enthused he was in that sporting atmosphere. I think Rohan saw a lot of his grandfather in Vivaan. His demeanour, his caring and sensitive nature, the way he already commands attention, even his physical appearance—as extended family members had pointed out.

I could understand how Rohan's illness had affected Vivaan because once, when I was trying to reassure the seven-year-old, he turned to me and said, 'Mommy, you keep saying Daddy will come home. He still hasn't. I don't think he is coming home.'

It shattered my heart to hear his innocent words.

I had every intention to show Rohan to Vivaan on one of the video-calls. He had made me promise. He asked on his birthday, again. But when I made the scheduled call, Rohan's eyes were closed. I could not bring myself to give Vivaan the phone. It would completely destroy him. He had started sleepwalking the past month and had just started talking to a therapist during the separation. 'Vivi, I promise you, I will show you Daddy when he wakes up fully. He is so tired right now.'

Vivaan walked away in a huff.

Krishna, who by then was coming over almost every day to babysit the trio when I was doing chores, had surprised us by renting a foam machine for the afternoon. While Texas was allowed to open businesses at 25 per cent capacity after weeks of a complete shutdown, the high number of cases was not reassuring. A new report had brought forth a discovery which was not pleasant— apparently, two American had died of coronavirus in early February, at least three weeks before the previously known first death in the country. Johns Hopkins had just two days before confirmed one million cases and counting in the country. It was too soon and too scary to have his school friends come over. But that did not stop many of his friends' parents stopping by and dropping off balloons and cupcakes at the porch, waving to the birthday boy from afar. He spent the day with his siblings and Krishna but I knew he was upset.

'I wish Daddy was here,' he told me, his forlorn face tugging at my heart. And while cutting the cake in the backyard, we had to literally coax him to do so. He kept refusing, throwing tantrums, walking away whenever Aria went up to him, pushing away Ayaan.

'Give it time, Manasi. It's expected. He is feeling a sense of loss and does not have a way to articulate it like adults,' Vasanti empathised that evening.

After the children were in bed, Vivaan still angry, I checked up on Rohan's update—the hospital had started intermittent dialysis and continued physical therapy. They wanted to ensure Rohan's body movements continued and got better with time. The duty doctor was candid: 'We need to get him moving. At this point, he is awake but isn't conscious of what he's gone through.'

In India, the stringent lockdown was continuing, extended for two more weeks. The announcement came on Vivaan's birthday. My parents were stuck at home. My mother had so far been successful in evading the police to go to her astrologer but worrying about her getting caught kept me awake at night. Besides, the number of cases was only growing and, at times, I didn't know who I should worry about more—my husband in hospital or my aging parents alone in a crazy world.

Rohan's cardiologist was extremely positive about his progress. After seeing him smile very slightly on FaceTime the next day, I was told he was going back to physical therapy, and his doctor took over. It was an infectious happiness because talking to the medical professional, I started to smile. 'We need to think of long-term care now. I have no doubt in my mind that Rohan can go home with some care. At this moment, I cannot comment on the tracheal tube. Maybe we have to remove it at a later date. But we shall get to that. Right now, we need to think of the obstacles he has overcome to open his eyes.'

I sighed for a second, and allowed my stressed out body to relax just a little. Then, we got around to discussing what he meant by long-term care. Long-term acute care hospitals (LTACHs) are facilities, usually inside an acute care hospital, where they primarily treat patients with serious medical conditions. These are patients who no longer need intensive care but still need more care than one can receive at home or a rehabilitation centre. In Rohan's case, it would be at LTACH that he would eventually be weaned off the ventilator after the ECMO machine came off. Prolonged dependency on ECMO can lead to formation of blood clots, even cause a stroke.

The day liquor stores in India re-opened, the media reported snaking queues, whether it was Uttar Pradesh or Kerala. My mother called to say her astrologer firmly said Rohan's recovery was on track. Along with the astrology checks, my parents had also begun to invite a group of priests home to chant and pray for Rohan's recovery every other day. All socially distanced, of course. It was now 4 May. On a happier occasion, Rohan would be foxing me with *Star Wars* references, even try and make the zwoosh sound like Luke Skywalker fighting Darth Vader. Unfortunately, Rohan was fighting another battle—to get back to breathing normally.

The doctors were by his bedside getting ready to perform a bronchoscopy procedure. They would look at the airways in his lungs using a lighted thin tube to check for any bacterial growth. I was nervous, despite many reassurances that this was one of the safest procedures. After the weeks of constant fear and routine procedures turning risky, I turned to faith. It was after Vasanti's guidance that my mind calmed. When I video-called him later, the nurse showed me Rohan's face and reported that the physical trainer had made him sit up. It was a sign that his body was beginning to recover. My focus was only on his eyes. They were still drowsy, fluttering to stay open. I don't think his brain was registering what was happening around him. I was not sure whether he realised how weak his body was. His heparin dosage had been increased as the ECMO setting was lowered.

That whole week, we just waited. Waited with bated breath for him to separate from ECMO. Every day, the goal seemed to get closer, with little nuggets suggesting it was going to be soon. He sat for five minutes by the side of the bed, after which he collapsed with tiredness and dozed off for some solid hours. His nurse tried to engage his cognitive function by constantly asking questions about his family. I had sent a laminated picture of the five of us along with some affirmations Vasanti had requested be put directly in front of Rohan. While the affirmations were talking to Rohan's soul, I was hoping constantly that seeing our images would aid his brain recovery, if at all he had lost any memory.

'When I pointed at you and asked the patient if he could recognise the person, you should have seen his face light up,' his nurse would say. Rohan still could not use his voice, it rasped when he tried; but his fingers were gaining dexterity. The nurse knew of his love of cricket and would switch to an old match on TV, hoping that hearing the commentary would help. 'He does seem happy hearing anything cricket. I was trying to understand the game but did not really get far,' his nurse laughed. It was her first time listening to cricket commentary and without Rohan's expert knowledge, she had no idea what was happening!

Dr Samar Sheth, his main cardiologist, was keeping up my spirits as I dealt with other mundane chores. 'We are sure Rohan can get off ECMO soon but first, we want to do a trial run.' Vasanti did not say no, and I gave my consent. Bhushan came to take the children to Austin on 7 May, so I could have some peace. I was physically recovered but now, I needed to get my professional life on track. I had to re-join work the following week on a part-time basis. My colleagues were more than understanding of the situation, offering regular prayers for Rohan.

The children had been cooped up at home for days on end but had been keeping busy drawing cards for their father. They would show me their brightly coloured, beautifully designed masterpieces, glittering in places. The cards always had a big red heart somewhere. I knew how much they missed Rohan's presence. They also chanted along with me when I prayed. I don't think they understood the mantras, but it made me feel at peace when they sat next to me daily as I said the affirmations. Their folded hands and closed eyes always cheered me up.

As the twins made their way to the car, Bhushan finally gave me a massive bear hug. 'Manasi, I don't have words to explain what this feels like,' he cried. I hugged him right back, and held on till Aria called out that it was going to get late. Bhushan wiped off a stray tear and looked around for Vivaan. He was at the front door, his stance stubborn, arms crossing his chest: 'I am not going.' He had made a decision and there was no changing his mind. He wanted to give me support during the upcoming Mother's Day weekend.

The trial run was conducted in the evening as Vivaan and I sat by the phone drinking hot chocolate. Rohan's ECMO setting was slowly lowered till his lungs were completely unsupported by the machine for a while. The hospital call reassured me that taking him off ECMO was a real possibility.

'When are we thinking of doing it?'

'Tomorrow,' Dr Sheth replied.

Vivaan hung around me all morning on Friday. Our respective parents were praying in Mumbai and Pune, Vasanti and Avinash were sending their healings connecting Rohan's soul, I was keeping calm by chanting mantras. Vivaan, beside me, had his eyes firmly shut. I know Sudha Mavashi and Ravi Mama were doing their bit. 'Let us hear Daddy's song, Mommy,' Vivaan said, turning up the laptop volume so the mantras, on loop, could be heard better. This was the day I was waiting with bated breath. I later realised he had been clutching a card he had made for Rohan throughout. It read, 'I Love u Daddy'.

My phone rang at 12.30 pm. Before I could say 'Hello', Dr Sheth's voice boomed, 'Manasi, it is out!'

The positive joy in his voice was unparalleled.

I blinked a couple of times. It had happened. Rohan was off ECMO. He was breathing; we had moved far away from the end-of-life protocol discussions in early April. I sent a silent prayer to Sai Baba and then asked, 'Are you sure?'

'Of course I am. I am standing next to Rohan and by god, the room looks huge without the machine.'

It really did. Rohan's bed and ventilator barely took up space, earlier dwarfed by the ECMO machine and various tubes keeping him alive. Now, while my mind was processing details over the video-call, I thought I heard the words 'move', 'real test' and 'heart'.

'Wait, what?'

'As I was saying, now starts Rohan's real test. We need to keep a close eye to see if anything untoward happens. Also, we will move him to a different unit because he no longer needs the ECMO nursing care,' Dr Sheth explained.

Vasanti sent me a warning text in the evening, before I dozed off: 'I think Rohan has a urine infection.'

Rohan was still asleep but at around 1 am, began to develop a fever. The hospital called later in the morning to give me the update. Rohan's body was so dependent on the ECMO machine to maintain a certain body temperature, that only now would the doctors realise his real bodily reactions. I peppered the caller with questions. 'Why does he have fever? 'Is it an infection? 'Is it a reaction to something?'

Rohan's bloodwork and urine samples were sent for analysis. But we had to wait till Monday for the reports. The labs could not send us details during the weekend, leaving me hanging. In the meantime, a broad spectrum of antibiotics was started to lower the fever. Despite trying, that weekend the doctors were unable to pinpoint where the fever stemmed from. It was a matter of concern but nothing that could deter Rohan's recovery.

Vivaan shook me awake Sunday morning. It was Mother's Day. He hugged me in bed and looked up with soulful puppy eyes. 'Mommy, can I talk to Daddy today?'

Rohan's voice was raspy, barely audible. He was mainly communicating with hand gestures. The moment he laid eyes on Vivaan over the video-call, the body language of both father and son changed. Vivaan was excited, just to be able to finally see his dad; Rohan's gestures became more animated. He ended the call with a flying kiss, the effort causing him pain. But Vivaan was over the moon. He finally believed his father would come home to him.

❧

The Long Wait

I had never wanted materialistic things for my birthday. When Rohan's condition became serious enough to question if he would survive the ordeal, one night, alone and still COVID positive, I asked Sai Baba for only one thing: 'Rohan has to wake up by my birthday. I do not care the condition he is in, but I want him alive and returned.'

Half my wish was granted but waking up alone on 29 May with the other side of the bed empty, felt hollow. The children were home, which was a relief and provided some sense of stability; the person I missed the most was Rohan. Yes, he was alive; the doctors felt his recuperation was in the right direction; but every day when I went to visit him in the progressive care unit (PCU), I could sense his dissatisfaction, his anger. Rohan's memory was fuzzy in parts and coupled with the tube still helping him breathe, he struggled to speak; I could understand how terrified he must feel.

As I sat in bed in the morning, my mind wandered to this day last year. There were balloons all over the house, the children had made posters and cards for me, Rohan had gotten me the most divine strawberry cake. So moist and flavourful, if I closed my eyes, I could still taste it.

I sighed with resignation. The happy memory was making me sad, as the joy was lacking a year on. Since we have been together, Rohan has always shown me in his own way how much he valued me. Every birthday, he would take me out to eat in places I had check-marked on my list, and bring me my favourite type of cakes. Something not too sweet, as Americans have teeth-clenching sugary desserts. I sighed again and got up from bed. I would quickly down a cup of coffee and then, head to Rohan. He would be waiting for me in his hospital room.

I left the children with a babysitter who had started coming in a week back. Kimberly was a god-sent. When doctors allowed me to visit Rohan, finding someone to look after the trio was hard. Though businesses in the state of Texas were opening up, the number of confirmed cases was not going down. Water parks had begun their operations with limited capacity on my birthday but the number of cases had crossed over 61,000. As if that was not worrying enough, two days prior Johns Hopkins University confirmed that this novel strain had killed more than 100,000 people across the country. Simply put, almost 900 people were dying each day since the first reported case. The world was sick and we were extremely lucky because Rohan was alive and awake. Finding childcare proved to be extremely difficult as word had spread far and wide that my children and I were affected by coronavirus.

'You say you are fine, but how do we know for sure?'

'Oh, you are that Manasi…no, sorry, I can't babysit your kids.'

'Coronavirus? Oh no, sorry.'

I had opted for full disclosure while searching for help. It was getting tougher to keep the three with Krishna every time I went to the hospital. He is in his seventies, so asking him repeatedly to look after the boisterous trio would be taking advantage of his kindness. Some days I left them with Kala aunty and Shekar uncle, who had taken it upon themselves to make sure we were doing alright, plying us with food and essentials since early May. On other occasions, I left them with our kind neighbour. Another neighbour suggested Kimberly's name to me. She is, in fact, the daughter of my old cleaning lady, who currently works at my friend's place. My friend inquired and the youngster immediately agreed.

'Are you sure?' I asked again. 'We have not had any luck so far because we have recovered from the virus but my husband is still in hospital.'

'Don't you worry about that. We are here for you, Mrs Manasi.' True to her word, Kimberly started work the very next day.

Kimberly's arrival was the cherry on the cake after a busy week. Looking after the three was her first babysitting job but it did not seem she lacked experience. From the first day, she became friends with the children and by the time my birthday came, Kimberly had them wrapped around her fingers.

Rohan looked better; his cheeks were flushed because of physiotherapy, but his eyes were angry. I did not expect Rohan to remember it was my birthday but what hurt me was his annoyance.

When he saw me enter, he looked away in a huff. When I coaxed him to look my way, he angrily turned and pressed his lips together. His eyes narrowed. He shook his right fist, and then pointed towards the door, mouthing, 'Go'. The tube in his throat was obstructing his speech but his gestures made his feelings clear.

I rushed out of the room before he could see me sobbing. I did not take his antagonism to heart but it hurt. I had gotten my wish, but it was an uphill battle before Rohan's independence, which he was craving, could return.

ಳಟ

'Will Daddy be able to play soccer? Can you ask him?'

It was 13 May, thankfully not a Friday. It had been two months since *the* sneeze. I had started working from home the previous day. It was initially stressful, but over the course of the day, I got used to it. I still could not believe that Bhushan and Priya had not missed a single day of work despite taking care of me and the children. Vivaan was busy kicking the ball around the backyard. I was getting ready to visit Rohan in the hospital. It would be the first time I would see him physically since he was hospitalised.

I was excited but also disheartened by the state of affairs. Thankfully, the reports were all fine so the presence of fever was disconcerting. Dr Sheth prepared me before I went inside the room. 'What you see over video may not be what you see in reality. You should be mentally prepared for that.'

His wise words made complete sense the moment I laid eyes on Rohan. His body had shrunk; his face was sunken making his eyes pop out but he looked better than during the first video-call; his toes, all ten of them, were completely black due to reduced blood supply; the ECMO machine was gone and only the ventilator and dialysis remained; the tube was still inserted in his trachea. It was not the Rohan who had left home almost two months ago.

The man in the bed smiled. I gingerly walked towards him, overwhelmed by the fact that he was alive. He was too weak to hold up his hand so I took his in mine. A shiver went down his spine. My mind could not register I was physically touching Rohan. I could not say a word for a while; we just looked at each other in complete silence. But we were speaking a language in our minds that connected us irrevocably at that moment.

I called both parents and Bhushan over video. Thank god for technological mercies.

My father waved at Rohan, my mother's tears flowed. Rohan's parents were trying to stay composed. Bhushan and Priya just stared, waiting for the situation to sink in. 'You look good, *beta*,' his mother mumbled, looking away from the video in case tears overwhelmed her composed nature. 'How are you, Rohan? How are you feeling?' my father asked. The atmosphere was so emotionally charged that despite wanting to reassure everyone he was fine, Rohan was unable to say a word. He tried, but after a couple of attempts, just nodded and smiled. I could see relief awash on all the faces on the video.

I had broken down a few times during the entire journey but at that moment, no tears flowed. I had promised myself I would cry next on the day Rohan was back to 100 per cent. He did not need my tears before that.

'Rohan.' He turned his face towards me from the call. 'Vivi wanted to know if you can play soccer with him. What should I tell him?'

He nodded, and then used two fingers of his dormant right hand to feebly make a gesture of someone running.

'So, do you promise?'

Rohan sucked in his breath. It was a deep breath. He was trying to muster all his energy to speak. I moved closer. And I finally heard his raspy voice, barely audible, say, 'Yes.'

I did not realise how much I had missed hearing his

voice, until I heard it after ages. He was back, and I knew, ready to fight to come home to play soccer with his son. That was a promise he intended to keep.

On 14 May, the day after I saw Rohan for the first time, he developed a rash on his left shoulder. While treatment started for the nasty redness, he developed a urine infection. Every day really epitomised what Dr Sheth had mentioned initially: 'One step forward, two steps back.'

Bhushan drove in with the twins on Saturday, 16 May. Being able to hug him once again lifted my spirits. Bhushan, later, confided that while everything was happening around us, one of the things that had affected him most emotionally was the inability to give me a hug when he knew that is what I needed. He carried with him more home-cooked Maharashtrian dishes Priya had packed, and after stepping back, looking at my face, made the decision to stay the night. 'I don't want you to be alone.'

The relief must have shown on my face because I cried out in happiness. It was the last day of Rohan's dialysis. The hospital was convinced his kidneys were functioning normally, without aid. The authorities had also decided he would soon be moved out of the intensive care unit to a PCU, the intermediary step before LTACH. In a PCU, patients still require a high level of skilled nursing but are far more stable than when in intensive care. Thus, the ratio of nurse-to-patient in PCU is more than in intensive care. Rohan's body scans the next two days did not show any anomalies so it seemed his recovery was finally on track. A wonderful indicator of progression.

As Rohan's strength slowly began to return, he was given an alphabet board to aid communication with staff, us, anyone really. I think Rohan was overjoyed with it at first. *Breaking Bad* is one of his favourite TV shows and he thought communicating with the board would be as cool as playing out the DEA scene in the show! However, the bothersome tube soon got the better of his excitement. Over the next two days, he would angrily gesture, his fingers curling up or extending at every answer I gave him. I was trying to put his mind at ease, trying to update him on everything that had happened, but a sanitised version. His eyes kept getting wider with each sentence but when he heard that I had brought his car back from Norfolk, he ran his hands through the air in distress, trying to ask me, 'Why?' I think he believed he could go back to Norfolk after he was discharged.

The effort to communicate tired him out. And the frustration grew. Often, he would just keep pointing to the alphabet 'F' on the board, to show how he was feeling. I knew him well enough to realise it was definitely an expletive he was indicating.

After some deliberation, it was decided that Rohan would be moved to the PCU in the same hospital on 20 May. So, the day before, I video-called both sets of parents when I went to visit him. Despite the dark circles under his eyes and sunken cheeks, the sight of Rohan brought smiles to their faces, a brief break from worry.

Both sets of parents were barely getting any sleep. They felt helpless, unable to do anything from so far away. The lockdown in the country had been extended till the end of the month; and it was also a cause for concern to know India had overtaken China in terms of the total number of cases reported. Just before the video-call, news channels had reported that India had crossed one lakh cases. Rohan did not know any of that, and with much determination, waved a short 'hello' to the screen. I could see the relief on the four faces. It was a brief moment, but a momentous occasion nevertheless.

His mother narrated an instance of Rohan's stubbornness after he dozed off. 'It is a relief that he is alive, but if only we could turn back time. If only he had gone to the hospital early…'

'It's okay, mom. He is fighting now.'

'I am so thankful for his fighting mentality,' she almost wept. 'His obstinacy goes both ways. I remember this one time when he was nine years old, playing a tennis match. He was losing but held on valiantly against a much older opponent. The referee postponed the match to the next day because the sun had set. He had a quiet stubbornness about him that night. He told me categorically that he would not give up. And he did not, pushing his opponent to the very edge. He finished runner-up, however. The tournament referee recognised his fighting spirit and much to everyone's surprise, awarded Rohan a special trophy. The trophy is still displayed in our living room. During this whole uncertainty, I keep looking at the trophy for strength, to help us guide through this turmoil.'

I was learning new stories about my husband.

I went to visit Rohan the day after his PCU move. It was a bright morning but as I stepped inside his new room, I could see annoyance writ large on his face.

'What happened?'

He just shook his head and gave me a brief smile.

Unlike intensive care, in the PCU, I could go and physically visit him every day. It felt like a blessing, to be honest. We had been apart before, but it was never a life-or-death situation. I did not care about all our disagreements, I had forgotten things that I disliked. I just wanted to be physically near him, touch his hand to make my mind believe he was truly awake. But it seemed Rohan was not enjoying his stay in the PCU from the very beginning. The low-grade fever that he had developed after getting off ECMO persisted and the doctors could not yet pinpoint the reason. The fever and his breathing tube were annoying him; it was only after much persuasion and coaxing did I realise that there was a possibility he was feeling neglected and was lonely.

The mild stroke he had suffered was also a matter of concern. Doctors had discovered some inflammation in his brain after a regular scan, and had mentioned that at this point, they only hoped things would improve with time. They hoped the stroke in his cognitive part of the brain would not affect his daily activities, but after experiencing such a severe trauma, a lot of thinking is abstract. Witnessing it from the outside, it felt Rohan was becoming forgetful, or his mind was wandering off in the middle of sentences. However, it was also heartening to receive messages from Vasanti, Sudha Mavashi and Ravi Mama assuring all of us that Rohan's condition was improving. I clung onto their words with hope.

A day before my birthday, I walked in to greet Rohan with a huge smile on my face to find him struggling to breathe. His eyes were wide, he was leaning forward trying to gulp in copious amounts of air but was unable to do so. I cried out just as a nurse entered.

'His heart rate had been fluctuating all morning.'

A normal resting heart should beat 60-100 times per minute. For an adult in his forties, the target heart rate zone should be 90-153. The predicted maximum heart rate should not exceed 180. Rohan's had been in a free-fall, ranging from 120-148 to 130-55.

'The cardiologist has been trying different medications to bring down the patient's heart rate under control.'

I looked at the laminated affirmations by the foot of his bed and closed my eyes to offer a prayer. When I opened my eyes, Rohan's terrified eyes greeted me. 'Home,' he mumbled with effort. 'Take...me...home.'

It took everything in my will power to reply in the negative.

'I can't, Rohan. You have to get better.'

That brief conversation must have played on Rohan's mind all night. I sensed his anxiety when I left, seeing him struggle had worried me immensely, but to see him gesture that I should go and leave him when I visited him the next day, the day I turned a year older, threw me off completely.

I burst into tears outside, sobbing softly so he could not hear. I knew he was not thinking straight but how could he believe that I did not want to take him home? How could he think that I wanted him to be at a medical centre when I wanted him home so we could celebrate together?

I drove home, my heart heavy and my mind aching with a dull throb. I just wanted to curl up under the covers. But I walked in to a surprise.

Kala aunty and Shekar uncle had come over with a cake and card. Krishna came with take-away food from an Indian restaurant. One look at my face, Krishna knew I was upset. 'Manasi, just be grateful that he is alive. He is improving.'

A honk outside made me look out the window and there was an ex-colleague of mine, waiting with a box in her hands. I was so shocked and delighted to see her after four years! Despite living in the same city, we do not always end up physically seeing each other. 'I got you *pav bhaji,* Manasi. I know you always loved it when I got it to office,' she said as she put the container on the driveway.

They all left by evening and the children were busy on their own, when I finally sat down with a cup of tea. I looked at a picture on the mantle. It was the five of us, dressed in fine clothes, smiling wide with excitement at the camera. It had been taken on our last trip to India. I shook my head. The memory seemed to belong to a past life.

The doorbell rang, I wondered who could that be. Lo and behold, opening the wooden door revealed Bhushan standing outside, holding a huge bouquet of flowers and a large cardboard box containing a home-baked carrot cake by Siya!

'Happy birthday, Manasi,' he gleefully showed his teeth, absolutely overjoyed that I had not been able to predict his surprise with my gut feeling. The children rushed out to greet their uncle, screaming, 'Bhushan, Bhushan!' Yes, the three believe Bhushan is their age, so they have never called him Mama or uncle, terms usually reserved for a mother's brother. And my brother has always been okay being their pal, playing along with their perception that they are all of the same age-group. Priya wished me over a video-call with Siya; then everyone sang as I cut into the cake. COVID-19 had ensured there was no blowing out of candles. I went to sleep with my heart light and headache gone but the sadness remained because I was missing Rohan's presence at the celebrations.

Bhushan, who had stayed over, came with me to the hospital the next morning. All this while, he had only seen Rohan over a video-call. I had seen him and Priya gulp to keep down their emotions, to stay strong in front of elderly parents. But there is a drastic difference between seeing him in person and looking at him over video. And just as Dr Sheth had prepared me, I explained scenarios he could be facing or sudden emotions he could be feeling when inside the room. Because of the virus, the PCU had a strict rule that only one visitor would be allowed per patient and it would have to be the same person to minimise contact and chances of outbreaks.

A special permission later, Bhushan went up alone as I waited in the car. A visitor is usually allowed inside a room for half an hour. I had checked the latest text from Vasanti and was about to respond, when I saw my brother rushing out. It had not even been ten minutes.

His eyes were brimming with tears and his heart was beating faster. I could hear his heartbeat in the quiet of the car. 'It was so painful, Manasi. I could not bear to see Rohan in that state,' he said, painfully uttering each word. 'How do you keep your emotions in check when you go to see him every day?'

He narrated that when he entered the room, Rohan's hand was bleeding as tests had just been completed. Due to his frail condition, in the few minutes that a nurse stepped outside to get some gauze, the part of the pristine white pillow that helped prop up Rohan, and on which his hand rested, turned crimson. 'I asked the nurse to change the pillow cover when she returned, told Rohan he was looking great and that he was going to fight this nonsense, and just ran down. I did not even wait for the elevator,' he said, trying to control the shaking that had overtaken him.

It was clear, as the days went by, that Rohan was not enjoying his stay at the PCU. If he could, he would walk out any moment. He felt the level of care at the ICU was better. The only time of day he was happy was when I was there. I could physically see his face droop if I peeked in after walking out the door. The doctors were still running brain scans to examine the stroke fallout and monitor bleeding. He was still on intravenous blood thinners but to move to the next step of his recovery regime, to the LTACH, he would have to take tablets orally. On the bright side, his ventilator settings were getting better, and being used only at night.

My communication with Vasanti, too, had increased considerably during this time. While initially, she would tell me to call from the room with Rohan's vitals, as the days progressed, she began to echo Rohan's feelings: a move away from PCU. Avinash had, in fact, emphasised the need to move Rohan to LTACH as soon as possible. He could sense Rohan's unhappiness continents away.

While approvals to move Rohan to long-term care were still pending, how could I simply ask the doctors to move him without any medical reason? 'They will not release Rohan, Vasanti, unless they are sure he can be moved,' I would counter, feeling utter helplessness at my inability to physically be there for Rohan through the day. However, there was a bright beacon of light at the PCU in the form of Rohan's respiratory therapist. She, too, was a clairvoyant and whenever on duty, would try to calm Rohan down, sensing his dissatisfaction.

As Rohan's strength recovered, the therapists tried to get him to be more physically active. One day, during physical therapy, a nurse lifted Rohan from the bed holding his armpits, and made him sit in a chair. Initially, he grumbled, aching from the move, but he managed to sit upright for an hour—much to everyone's surprise, including Dr Sheth. He was so buoyed by this step, he called me in the middle of my work calls to share his happiness. 'He is sitting, he is sitting,' he gleefully said. 'This is unbelievable.' Hearing the hopefulness emulating from Dr Sheth was a relief, I felt my body float with positivity.

But the euphoria came crashing down the next day. Rohan needed surgery. A simple vascular plug, but just the thought of him going under the knife again was disconcerting. There were fistula formations near Rohan's shoulder and this plug would effectively help in separating the vein from the artery. The procedure would be minimally invasive. The fistula could have been an after-effect of ECMO. I gave the go-ahead but something felt off. I could not think of any reason to refuse consent.

Before the procedure was conducted, however, the pulmonologist located a patch on Rohan's chest. They assumed it was a vessel rupture but they had no answer as to how it happened. I was informed the patch was not life-threatening in anyway but there was a possibility it would increase pressure in his blood vessels in the future, maybe causing them to rupture. I wish this was the end to my feeling of impending doom but no, the next few days were torturous.

'The patient is feeling extremely uneasy and has chest pain,' the nurse called to inform. I immediately leapt to conclusions but the staff told me Rohan might be just feeling uncomfortable after the procedure; his test results were all fine. The reason Rohan was weaned off the ventilator before he could be moved to LTACH was why he was at the PCU. Thus, usually, during the day, a CPAP (continuous positive airway pressure) machine was being used, shifting to the ventilator only at night. What CPAP does is deliver pressurised air through a hose and mask into the airway. The CPAP usage was increasing over the days, until one day they used it for eighteen hours. I was on my way to the hospital the day after, when a call came in.

'Rohan is asking for you.'

I pushed hard on the accelerator to reach him quicker.

Rohan was looking pale. His oxygen level had dropped to 50 per cent. I stood in the doorway looking in as doctors tried everything to get the oxygen level up. I had been hungry but looking at his face, my pangs were gone. I suddenly felt dehydrated, dizzy. I have lost count but I must have been there for hours when visitors are usually allowed for only thirty minutes. I finally had to leave at 6:30 pm, but his oxygen level was still not back up completely. They presumed Rohan could have pneumonia in his still-fragile body.

Vasanti and Avinash kept reassuring me throughout that Rohan was fine although the PCU was not good for his recovery progress. 'There will be ups and downs, but he is getting better.' I believed them, however hard it was because of medical results showing otherwise. I trusted them because I could see indicative changes when they chanted. To give you some examples, Avinash would often be on the phone when I visited Rohan. If his vitals were not great, Avinash would instruct me to keep my hand on Rohan's chest and chant after him. Within seconds I would see Rohan's heart rate and blood pressure on the monitor stabilise. Or when he explicitly told me to make a few changes around the house—remove a few posters and frames, put up printed mantras in specified directions—I could sense Rohan feeling better when I visited. Avinash was also absolutely certain Rohan would be off dialysis by a certain date. 'Call me on 16 May,' he had told Vasanti the day Rohan came off ECMO. Vasanti called on the specified date to confirm what Avinash already knew—Rohan would no longer need dialysis. They were all steps in the positive direction.

It was Avinash who asked Vasanti to reach out to Bharat when Rohan's oxygen level dramatically dropped. Vasanti had come across Bharat, a priest, randomly on a bus but had felt a healing energy radiating from him. Bharat's strict instruction for me going forward was to draw out all negative energies that were around Rohan. He would ask me to complete simple tasks like keeping a piece of ginger in a transparent container behind Rohan's bed. I would have to change the ginger piece every week but he assured it would be a boon in Rohan's recovery. (I kept doing it till Rohan left LTACH, and I firmly believe that aided in bringing Rohan home.)

Rohan was back on the ventilator full time on 7 June. It felt like a complete 360-degree turn from all the progress we had made. He needed a unit of blood because his haemoglobin count was low. Bhushan and I were alternately calling every couple of hours asking for updates. It was about 9 pm, when I had just made a cup of herbal tea and sat down to meditate in the living room that Bhushan rang. 'Manasi,' his voice shook. 'Rohan has tested positive.'

The calm I was attempting to maintain shattered. Rohan was close to being moved to the LTACH, for which he needed to test negative. This result would undo everything. I cried to Vasanti for guidance, panicking though I was trying hard not to. Vasanti, calm as always, heard me out and then took a deep breath.

'He has tested negative.'

'What?' In my mind I replayed Bhushan's message that Rohan had tested positive.

'There was a mix-up, yes,' she said, her voice so far away. 'Just wait for two days and you'll see.'

I believed her because I had faith in her affirmations, although it was tough to stay calm in the middle of this calamity. Bhushan offered to come down but I felt it would not do anyone any good.

I could not see Rohan in person because of the positive reading. But I dropped off a phone with the COVID ICU nurses. When I had gone through Rohan's belongings after picking them up from ER, his inbox and voicemail was flooded with messages of concern. I put it away in his bedside drawer and picked up an old mobile lying in storage. It was so old that it could only be used for messages and calls but for the present purpose, it was perfect. I got a new number issued that morning and put it in the phone. I knew Rohan would be tempted to go online and it was not fruitful given his state. There were too many articles floating on the internet about his condition. He was already depressed about the PCU and reading the articles could have an adverse effect. But now, with a phone in his proximity, he would be closer to his family—he could text whenever he wanted. The duty doctor's words provided some moral support—'Rohan is clinically not declining and it also does not feel he is positive.'

Rohan had been immediately transferred to the COVID unit after testing positive and the doctors, despite the move, did a second plug surgery. I knew it would be painful, but it was also what he needed to get better. An email that came to my inbox also kept me motivated. It read that once Rohan tested negative, he would be immediately moved to LTACH. I heaved a sigh of relief.

I called the hospital early on 10 June. I had not been able to sleep all night. I was on tenterhooks. When the nurse took the call, something in her voice, just the way she said 'Hello', filled me with hope. And then she uttered the words that I received with shaky laughter and tremendous relief. 'Rohan has tested negative.'

I persuaded the medical staff to not move Rohan back to the PCU while we arranged his transfer to LTACH. Now, it was all about navigating the mountains of paperwork to get formal clearance for the transfer, working in tandem with insurance.

The staff helped me as for the next two days, Rohan was kept at a different ICU. On the morning of 12 June, official approval for the move to LTACH came through. I hugged Vivaan, who was sitting beside me, playing with an action figure. 'Daddy is going to move!'

Vivaan got excited. 'Is he coming home?'

My eyes gleamed with joy as I mentally danced around the room.

'He is very close to coming home, honey. Very close.'

Some Care But Not Enough

The move to LTACH was the next step to bringing Rohan home. After the ordeal our family had gone through, I wanted to be sure they had the necessary care facilities to treat him, if things went awry. I do understand that LTACH does not necessarily have ICU nurses and staff who are trained for emergencies. I wanted to be mentally at peace before Rohan took another ambulance ride. All my queries tumbled out:

'Do you check bloodwork every day?'

'Rohan has A+ blood type. Do you have it in stock?'

'Do I have to arrange for blood if you do not?'

I could visualise the stunned face of the LTACH staff with whom I was speaking. It could have been bemusement, one can barely make out over the phone.

'No one has ever asked us these questions,' he finally answered.

That immediately annoyed me. 'What if Rohan's oxygen level drops and he is unable to ring for the nurse?' I countered, ready to take on another verbal fight. But I bit down other arguments, steadied my voice, and tried to ensure Rohan would have access to emergency care, if required. 'I will make sure if you need blood for Rohan, you will have it.'

An ambulance ride is always scary. It conjures images of the unknown, of things that could go wrong. When Rohan left home in an ambulance in March, the wail of sirens that broke the still of that night is still fresh. The sirens awoke the children and they came down to hug me because they were scared. They had never heard the sound outside their home. How alone Rohan must have been through that ambulance ride, without a familiar face in sight. Did he feel nervous? Was he frightened? But this time round, he would not be alone. I promised him that when I texted him after the LTACH move was approved.

The ambulance did not look quite as menacing when I stood in front of the vehicle. Rohan was prepped by the hospital staff and taken through long corridors to the dock where I waited. He looked so frail in the bed that carted him but I saw him smile once he saw I was there as promised. His tired eyes lit up for a brief second, before he slumped back and heaved. Even this tiny exercise had fatigued him. I sat by the ambulance driver while a paramedic kept vigil on Rohan's oxygen level in the back. It was a 15-minute ride but it felt longer. The drab evening sky did not help either, combined with the charged atmosphere of the institution we were leaving, everything around us dark and sombre. I felt I was playing a tiny part in one of Carlos Ruiz Zafon's Gothic Spanish novels because the oppressive atmosphere reeked of death. Yet there we were, moving towards the light.

The ambulance driver must have seen my trepidation because he tried to lighten the mood. 'Hey, there. I think we turned off the oxygen, dude,' he joked. I burst out laughing, the veil of heaviness slipping away. He had made an exception for us as no family member was allowed to ride in an ambulance with a patient during the pandemic.

As I wiped away the laugh tears, the topic changed to the coronavirus cases. 'Your husband is lucky, dude. Really lucky.' I did not have to be told that twice. Luck, determination, prayers—they had all played a part in Rohan leaving the hospital alive. This good fortune had not smiled on many, many other COVID patients. Just two days before, Texas had hit a new daily high with over 2,000 new cases added to almost 80,000 across the state. Cases had soared in states like Arizona and Florida which had rushed to open the economy. Johns Hopkins had just confirmed that the USA had crossed two million confirmed cases. My parents mentioned, in one of our calls, that India was beginning to reopen her economy in phases, despite soaring numbers. On 12 June, the day Rohan was being transported to LTACH, India had officially become the fourth worst COVID-hit country with over three lakh cases.

'Maybe we just move to New Zealand, eh?'

I nodded in agreement and jokingly said, 'I need to start to look for a job there.' The world had heard the New Zealand Prime Minister announce some days earlier that the island nation had no active cases.

Rohan was dozing off by the time we reached the destination. I went up with him to see the room after taking special permission because visiting hours were over. Everything seemed satisfactory, I waved goodbye from the door after setting up the affirmations and family pictures. Rohan was already asleep, a hint of a smile on his face.

ೞ

Our goal at this LTACH facility was to wean Rohan off the ventilator, getting him to breathe normally without external support. To get his muscles stronger, for him to speak better with therapy, and importantly, to get him on a solid food diet. Dr Sheth had prepared me mentally for the long haul but I couldn't help wishing for faster progress.

The room Rohan was assigned at LTACH was big and airy, a huge window looking out to blue skies if he turned his head sideways. It was a big change from the previous hospital room. All these establishments have pristine white walls and a sterilised atmosphere, so a window through which one can look out makes all the difference.

I was allowed to visit him every day for one hour only. The children wanted to see their father, especially Vivaan who would question me daily. Unfortunately, LTACH would only allow one regular visitor with no exceptions for any children under the age of ten. They were extremely strict on that count. They were so strict, that come the end of the 60-minute mark, guards would walk in and firmly escort me out. This happened almost every day because I always overstayed the hour, with Rohan imploring me to stay back five more minutes. The guards and I actually worked out an unspoken system—they would tell me time was up, then go along the corridor and round up other visitors before coming back to Rohan's room right at the end. This gave us about seven additional minutes together. After what we had been through, I did not want to leave his side even for a minute. Once, I even told him he could eat dinner in front of the television set as much as he wanted after he was home!

The staff were planning on putting in a speaking valve to aid Rohan's speech. The one-way valve is attached to the opening of the tracheostomy tube. The valve opens when breathing in oxygen and closes when breathing out, allowing the air to flow up through the vocal cords for sound to emit. Thus, in short, the patient can breathe out through the mouth and nose instead of the tube. It takes time to adjust to the valve, and I was told Rohan's case depended on his ability to get used to it. Speech therapy had already begun for him. I had gotten used to him trying to talk during his hospital stay but it had taken me time to understand the nuances once he stopped using the alphabet board. His speech therapist at the LTACH was focusing on assessing his cognitive functions related to producing voice in different situations, including other motor skills and swallowing capabilities.

It was a Sunday morning when the valve was put in. Kimberly did not work on weekends and my Saturday babysitter Jessica, another god-sent who had contacted me through a Facebook group, was unable to offer her services that Sunday. With my babysitters coming regularly during the week, either Krishna or Kala aunty kept watch on Sundays when I went to visit Rohan. This particular Sunday, Krishna volunteered to come by and keep the three company. 'We'll have fun, don't worry. Just think of what you want to say to Rohan when you meet him,' he said.

I drove to the facility in a state of excitement, my heart thumping. I knew the valve would not dramatically improve Rohan's speech overnight, but I could not help think that maybe, he would be more articulate. My nerves were jumpy like on a first date, which was a complete contrast to our actual first date in Pune. 'Calm down,' I told myself as I went up the elevator. Speaking to Vasanti the night before had also helped, when she reaffirmed that the valve would be beneficial for Rohan.

There he was, sitting upright against the pillows. He was waiting for me. The valve was covered with a white covering; it protruded from near his throat. The nurse had taken me aside just as I entered the corridor to let me know Rohan's vocal cords may be affected when speaking because of the valve. His breathing pattern, too, may change, though at the moment he was doing well. Rohan was usually clean-shaven but today he had a stubble. On the whole, he looked well.

'How are you?' I held my breath, waiting for his answer.

There was a delay as Rohan tried to breathe in. Then, taking all the time in the world, he whispered more loudly than before, 'I…want…ice cream.'

I was shocked. Eyes wide, mouth agape under my mask, I could not believe my ears. Here I was waiting for him to tell me *something* about us, anything about missing me or the children. I would even have been happy if he had just taken my name. But ice cream? Really? The man's first words to me after getting the valve which would help his speech, was to reinforce his insane love for cold dairy? I don't think I was this shocked when it finally dawned on me that Frankenstein was the last name of the fictional scientist by Mary Shelley, and not the name of the monster he created during an English class in school. Nor when Darth Vader revealed he was, indeed, Luke's father.

Rohan's swallow test came up soon. Since March, he was being fed intravenously. But if he could eat on his own, it would be a step closer to his release. The minor stroke he had suffered was still being monitored and the swallow test was a procedure to check for dysphagia. When eating, the food travels from the mouth into the pharynx, then through the oesophagus to the stomach.

This motion is aided by various muscles along the way. Similarly, a flap called the epiglottis blocks food particles from entering the lungs when breathing. If one cannot swallow food and breathe, or face severe difficulty while doing so, it can effectively lead to problems like aspiration. But Rohan passed the exam with flying colours.

I had brought him homemade mango milkshake, thick and frothy, to celebrate this much-deserved victory. The nurse later told me he weakly managed only three or four spoonfuls. Then it dawned on me that it was the first food Rohan was taking orally since 24 March. I felt a sense of sudden shock, promising myself I would always be ready to make mango milkshake for Rohan whenever he wanted them in the coming months, even if I had to go to a tropical country to get the best fruit!

After all the bodily damage, he had completely lost his appetite, a U-turn from always wanting to snack. 'It will get better, this is just the first step,' the nurse said.

I video-called Rohan's colleague Ranit in Norfolk during the week. Rohan is extremely close to him and treats him like a brother and through all this, Ranit was kept updated on his friend's condition. He was, initially, the only one in the office to know. I knew he was anxious the last two months because he would text me every week asking questions. He had confided to me, before Rohan woke up, how every time I said there was no progress, a part of him would be crushed. When I texted to give him a heads up, that Rohan was strong enough for a call, his happiness was unbound.

They smiled at each other at first but I could see the shock on Ranit's face, even though he tried to compose himself. I could see a visible improvement in Rohan because I was meeting him almost every day, but for someone who has not been in contact since the hospitalisation, Rohan's physical features would be a surprise. He had lost so much weight, which he never would have even with a balanced lifestyle. The valve jutting out gave him an extraordinary appearance. And by then, he had a full beard, refusing to allow them to shave him. The man in the hospital bed barely bore a resemblance to Rohan as people knew him.

'Everyone misses you,' Ranit said. And then reassured Rohan that everything at work was fine. All projects were on track, Rohan did not have to worry. All he had to concentrate on was improving so he could go home. He held up a document on the screen which had messages wishing Rohan and us well from all his teammates, bosses and friends at Norfolk. The gesture was so sweet, I could sense Rohan getting emotional without saying much. I, too, was overwhelmed. I must have done something good sometime in my life to be blessed by such generosity from people I did not know.

By the time I left that evening, Rohan was at peace. He waved bye with a smile.

CRED

Rehabilitation was on at full speed. I had left some books, including a biography of Sachin Tendulkar, by his bedside. The affirmations and family pictures were always next to him, and Vasanti, my parents, even my distant relatives were sending him healing thoughts at different times of the day. My daily schedule was set by then— work from home in the morning, do my chores, visit Rohan with homemade food, then at night, meditate and chant when the world was quiet.

However, Rohan was not in a good mental state at LTACH. He felt lonely. At the hospital, the care was specialised but here, he was alone in a lovely room right at the end of a corridor. He had no one to talk to except for the nurses and doctors who came to check on him or aid in his recovery. The nurses also discouraged him from ringing the call bell for every little thing. He confided that the only times he felt hopeful was during my visits. How long can one look out the window or read a book in such a state? Watching the news was not uplifting either. He would get further depressed because the news highlighted marches and vigils for the late George Floyd, whose untimely death had mobilised communities across the country. The headlines would also scream big bold numbers of confirmed COVID cases and deaths.

Rohan would be asked to sit beside his bed every morning and evening to strengthen his core. Even stretching his arms was a task at the beginning; the more he practised, the easier it became. He then progressed to sitting on a chair for some minutes before that became an hour or two. Then, he was slowly made to walk with a walker and help, a few steps at a time, until one day the physical therapist proudly said Rohan had walked 92 feet! The news seemed unbelievable. Rohan would text me every day the number of steps he had walked and I would reply with more encouragement. The same day he was also able to do more leg presses than before. His speech, too, was improving: he was able to enunciate shorter sentences without breaking to gasp for air. He was able to have soup and pasta in a few days, and then progressed to the soft mushy *khichdi* or *dal-chawal* I would get for him. On some days, he would merrily have ice cream, ignoring healthy food but I could not stay mad at him for long. He deserved a break too.

One fine day, one of Rohan's nurses called to say the doctor was going to reduce his tracheal tube size. I leapt with joy; it meant things were falling into place. However, by then, another issue had crept up. It was expected but Rohan thought everything was falling apart.

Some patients are able to go home from LTACH. It is a myth that patients admitted in long-term care are required to stay there for a minimum of 25 days. The amount of time depends on the complications or injuries, and the LTACH staff usually creates individual plans for each patient. In Rohan's case, the doctors mentioned, which Bindu had told us earlier, that he would be sent to a rehab centre before being allowed to go home. LTACH had aided in recovery but he was not in a good enough shape to be discharged. I said okay but was not willing to compromise on the rehab centre he would be moved to. I had done my due diligence—the best in the country, if not the entire world, was right here in Houston. A 134-bed state-of-the-art rehab and research hospital that focussed on patients with great care and did everything possible to make the transition easier.

The day I got a call from the specified rehab centre, I felt as if Rohan's time in medical institutions was shortening. But, as usual, there was an initial snag. A LTACH representative tried to convince me Rohan would receive similar care in any other rehab centre. I refused; it was the premier institute or none at all. I do not, to this date, understand why she kept insisting on moving Rohan despite my disapproval. But once the specifics were sorted, it was time to get Rohan ready for the final move in a week's time.

Rohan, however, was under the impression he would be heading home from the LTACH. One of his doctors had inadvertently mentioned during a check-up that he would be 'getting out of here next week.' He had obviously referred to the rehab centre move. In Rohan's mind, this meant he was going home. If he could jump with excitement, he would have but in his condition he could only showcase his enthusiasm with smiles. His eyes widened with disbelief when I told him about the rehab centre.

'No,' he said, shaking his head.

'You have to. The rehab centre is to help you get better. It will help you come home.'

His brows scrunched together in a scowl, he crossed his arms across his chest and kept shaking his head, refusing to listen to anything further from me. His eyes then narrowed. He clenched his fists. His body trembled, not in fear but seething anger. I had never seen Rohan this angry in all the years we have been together.

'You…don't want me…to…come home,' he said with his jaws clenched, the pain pronounced in each word he uttered.

I stared at him, hurt by his accusation. 'I fought for you, Rohan. How can you say that?' I quietly answered.

Rohan would not calm down. The head-shaking had gotten so vigorous I thought he would get dizzy. His fists were still clenched tight. His cheeks were getting redder every second.

I did not want his heart rate to jump. So I walked away, hoping my leaving would calm him. There was no point arguing with a man who would not listen to reason, or did not possess the capability at that time because of the long-drawn recovery process.

I slammed my car door shut, breaking the surprising quiet of the parking garage. I was hurting, too. A solitary tear slid down my cheek. I brushed it away, pursed my lips, and determination flooded through me. Rohan was going to the rehab centre whether he liked it or not. Because that was the only way our family could finally be reunited after months of separation.

The Last Battle

I woke up on 2 July with hope in my heart. As I lay in bed, comfortable under the duvet, my mind went back to the disastrous day when Rohan left in the ambulance. It felt like forever though it had been only three months. I was tired, my body needed physical rest. I wanted to curl up under the covers and sleep. But I could not, not yet at least. The last stage of the fight was pending, starting that evening.

Ayaan and Aria came running to my bedroom squealing with delight. Watching them rush in made me break into a smile. It was their fifth birthday. And for a moment, they had forgotten all the gloom surrounding our family. Aria, though she stays in her own world, is much attached to Rohan, while Ayaan is more of a

Mama's boy. Rohan would often tease him that Ayaan wanted my help with everything. Ayaan would loudly protest, 'No, Daddy,' and they would continue the back and forth teasing until Ayaan collapsed with laughter in Rohan's arms. These past months had been terrible for the two. They were too young to be going through such an ordeal.

During their visits to Bhushan's home in Austin, the twins would run wild, expressing their joy freely in the backyard. Bhushan had recently added a dog to his family. A stray had suddenly showed up one day, and stuck by his side. The search for its owners having led nowhere, Ginger had become a beloved family member in a short time, much to the twins' delight. The last time the twins were in Austin for a weekend, they did not leave Ginger alone for a minute, and the dog lapped up all the attention.

'Mommy, when can we eat cake?' Aria asked, looking up at me from under the covers. 'Very soon,' I said. Ayaan did not say anything, just hugged me tighter. Maybe he felt an uneasiness, maybe he knew I would be away for most of the celebrations in the evening.

Rohan was going to be moved to the rehab centre at 5 pm. Kimberly had put up a birthday banner in the kitchen, Krishna had come bearing gifts, and I got the cake set up just before leaving for LTACH. I hoped things would go smoothly; paperwork can take a notoriously lengthy amount of time as I had figured out dealing with hospitals these few months.

I could sense Rohan's excitement at leaving LTACH. I think, after he had calmed down, he was able to come to terms with the reality that faced him. He realised he was not in a condition to go home and would need more strength. The therapists at LTACH had mentioned that Rohan's attitude had changed in the past week; there seemed to be a fire lit inside because he was throwing himself with everything he had into any kind of therapy. He was pushing himself to do better. He had tested negative for the virus twice in a row—a prerequisite for the move.

The tracheal tube that had been part of Rohan's body for two months had to be removed prior to his transfer to the rehab centre. The back and forth with the LTACH representative and my determination to get him to the best facility the city offered had left me emotionally drained. But that was behind us, and now one had to look ahead. The staff removed the tube that very afternoon when Rohan was to leave. The removal went off with ease and Rohan was relieved that he was at a stage where he did not require it any longer. All the hard work he had been doing was paying dividends.

I waved to Rohan as the staff brought him down to the waiting ambulance. There was no trace of fear or fatigue. I understood what the doctors meant, something had changed in Rohan. Unlike the last ride we took together, this time I was allowed to sit beside him in the back along with a paramedic. The ride was only five minutes, thankfully the paperwork releasing him did not take long, Rohan holding my hand throughout. 'Wish Ayaan and Aria. Tell them I will be back soon,' he said, still whispering but getting better each day.

I was pleasantly surprised. Rohan's cognitive thinking was getting better though there were lapses. The LTACH nurses had mentioned he would sometimes doze off in the middle of sentences or forget names of mundane objects, trying to describe what he needed. Still, I was positive about the outcome. I knew our healing affirmations were helping, as were Sudha Mavashi and Ravi Mama's healings. Plus Avinash, Vasanti and Bharat's powers. My mother's astrologer was also sure of Rohan's recovery. A group of friends who chanted the '*Mahanmritanjay*' mantra for Rohan every day virtually supplemented all the prayers from extended family and strangers. And, I knew Sai Baba was keeping a watch over him. We had all the time in the world.

⌘

The rehab centre is one of the best in the country. They have interdisciplinary treatment teams that help a patient get ready to go home. From cognitive and communication therapy to mobility skills, pool therapy to playing sports, the teams formulate an individualised healing plan for a particular patient. I was told I too would have family training days to make sure I was ready to receive Rohan and make sure he was doing well once he was home. The pep talk was great; however, once we started the admission process, there was a hitch. I was wishing, just for once, that the transition would be smooth but I guess it was not in the stars.

'What do you mean he will be in a semi-private room? This most certainly was not conveyed to me.'

I was literally trying to hold back from lashing out at the rehab centre representative.

'We are sorry, but no private rooms are available.'

The room Rohan was allotted already had another patient, the beds separated by a thin curtain. The poor man in the other bed was retching and coughing loudly.

'Rohan can't be in the same room as this man.' I was livid by this point and firmly but politely made it clear how insane the proposal sounded. 'Do you have any idea how vulnerable he is at the moment? He has just recovered from coronavirus, the after-effects are still lingering, and you seriously want to put him in a room with a man who is coughing, no offence to the patient?'

Confirmed cases in the state were so bad recently that lawmakers in New York mandated that travellers from Texas who went up north had to be quarantined for a fortnight. The European Union's list of fourteen countries from which travellers were allowed did not include the USA because it was not yet a 'safe country'. I mean, for heaven's sake, Texas's positivity rate stood at 10.24 per cent, a level last seen in mid-April under the Governor's stay-at-home order. And mask-wearing was non-negotiable. Just hearing someone cough or sneeze had become scary.

'But the other patient does not have the virus,' the representative reasoned. I was flabbergasted by the counter-argument. What was going on?

I took a deep breath to calm my nerves.

'If I had known you did not have a private room, I would not have brought my husband to your institution. If this is an insurance matter, if you think our insurance will not be able to cover the expenses of a private room, I will pay out of my pocket. But Rohan will only be in a private room,' I said, firmly.

I checked on Rohan, who looked tired. He was dozing a bit, and I let him. He had had a long day. I waited, tapping my foot against the tiled corridor nervously. The administrator came back and said a vacant semi-private room was available but there was no guarantee the bed would not be filled up.

'No, he needs a private room.' I was not going to budge.

After what seemed like hours of back and forth, there was some good news. Rohan was first moved to a semi-private room where the second bed was occupied by a brain-dead patient for a few hours before they were ready to move him to an isolation room. But 'The patient needs to be tested again. If negative, we will move him.'

'What are you talking about? He has two consecutive negative tests from the LTACH. We were allowed to move here because of that!'

The administrator stood his ground; unless Rohan was tested, he could not be moved to the big private room. I was at my wit's end dealing with this as Kimberly kept sending me pictures of the birthday I was missing.

'Let them do the test, Manasi. It will be negative,' Vasanti calmed me down from India.

I turned to the administrator and said, 'Okay, but you have to guarantee that once Rohan is moved to a private room, he will under no circumstances be moved out.'

They agreed.

It was close to midnight when Rohan was tucked in bed in his private room. It was a massive room with a large window. The walls were white, but in the darkness of the night did not look ominous. Rather, it felt serene, like the calm after a storm.

By the time I reached home, the twins were tuckered out. Krishna was still waiting and Bhushan had surprised the duo coming from Austin with gifts and balloons. 'They were so happy, they ate so much cake that they probably crashed because of the sugar rush,' Bhushan laughed.

I showered and went to their rooms. They were both asleep, lost in a dreamy haze. I kissed them goodnight, vowing to make a family day once Rohan came home.

Finally, Krishna, Bhushan and I ate a hot dinner at 1 am. Steaming *idli-sambar*, the humble breakfast food, was all the nourishment I needed to end the day on a high.

ॐ

It took a day or two for the staff to set a routine for Rohan. Physical therapy, speech therapy and everything else they needed to do for Rohan to get fit. I think, after a few days, Rohan felt less anxious. He was definitely enjoying his stay at the rehabilitation centre more than LTACH or the PCU. The fact that his speech was getting better helped immensely because he could have conversations. In LTACH, he had no one nearby, but here, he developed a friendly bond with his therapists. He hated being pushed to do the exercises because his body hurt, so the therapists used positivity to motivate him. In fact, in just two days, he was able to get up and walk from his bed to the wheelchair without any help, much to our delight.

This one time when I was speaking with him, Rohan had just finished a round of physical therapy. He complained, 'Do you know, I asked him to give me my shoes because my legs were paining. But he was like, "No, you can walk. Get them yourself." I was so annoyed.'

I made a silly face, 'It is for your benefit only. The more you push, the faster you come home!'

'Yes, yes,' he agreed, rolling his eyes. I laughed aloud, because our banter seemed so normal. Something unimaginable for three long months.

I could not visit Rohan physically at the rehab centre, but unlike the past hospital stays, we were constantly connected over phone calls and messages. His dexterity was improving with time. We constantly texted, sending each other funny memes or just asking about mundane things; it felt like we were dating, just thirteen years too late! The technology did help, there is something to be said about constant gratification, unlike the weekly calls of the late 1990s. Rohan would make sure to do a FaceTime call before he dropped off to sleep by 8 pm. The therapists were keeping him busy to tire him out early. On most nights, the children would come on the call, shouting with excitement because they could see their dad on the screen. Rohan's face would light up when Aria and Ayaan fought for the phone, both trying to out-talk each other.

Vivaan would come after the twins finished their fight and discuss the latest moves he had practised in the backyard. 'Daddy, don't forget your promise. We have to play soccer when you are back,' he would remind Rohan. 'By Christmas, I will beat you,' Rohan would tease him.

Rohan also called his parents and mine. Seeing him slowly recovering gave them some peace of mind. His parents were still evading the police to violate the lockdown and go to the nearby temple to offer prayers. My parents continued their chants and affirmations. Dark circles were visible under their eyes; they said the same about me. Confirmed cases in India were still rising, it had recently become the third-worst hit country in the world with almost seven lakh cases. But there was also some semblance of good news because India, too, had joined other countries in the race to create a vaccine by agreeing to clinical trials. On the flip side, WHO's acknowledgement that there was 'evidence emerging' of the airborne spread of the virus besides transmission through respiratory droplets was definitely not a comforting thought.

Rohan's eating habits had improved, he was slowly progressing from mush to semi-solids and then, to more robust food. Every day, I drove to the rehab centre before my work started to drop off a carefully packaged food container. I really did not want to subject him to bland hospital food again. Rohan's appetite was returning but he still had a long way to go. I wanted to surprise him with one of his favourite foods, motivate him to push harder. Some days, I would put an *aloo vada* with his *khichdi*. He would immediately text with smiley emoticons when he opened the container at lunchtime. It still baffles me how much can one person love *aloo vada*. He would relish my *sabudana khichdi, aloo paratha, idli*s, eagerly waiting for his prize of good home food after a morning of therapy. His eyes would go wide with excitement when the staff brought the sanitised container to his bedside.

I would earlier scoff at films or television shows that portrayed a couple sending cute messages to each other. Now, I had started adding cute love messages with each of the containers. I wanted him to feel loved after everything he had been through. It made me feel good knowing he would read my message as he slowly savoured the food.

Everything was going well until one fine morning when I went to drop off hot *pav bhaji* without the usual oodles of butter for Rohan's lunch when a new guard stopped me. 'Sorry, ma'am. We cannot allow outside food.'

'This is blessed food. My husband cannot eat anything else,' I said, presenting a serious face. And that was all it took for him to relent—just the mention of faith.

Faith is such a powerful tool. My conviction in the divine had gotten firmer. I believed Vasanti, Avinash, Sudha Mavashi and Ravi Mama's healings, Bhushan's inputs, my family's mantras, even the children's prayers; they all played a huge role in helping Rohan out of the abyss. Medicines, yes, but one cannot deny the intervention of a supreme power. I had even begun to use simple affirmations to heal my grandmother in Denver whose health had taken a turn because of the changing weather.

After about ten days of Rohan's admission, I physically went inside to meet the staff for a family training day. I knew things would be different after Rohan was discharged, but talking to the staff made me realise how much things would have to change. The staff were doing everything in their power to make sure Rohan would be independent, albeit with some unavoidable modifications. During therapy, they were helping in strengthening his mobility skills, where he would be able to move on his own from the bed to the bathroom, to climb stairs with aid, to eat and dress himself, and more. I, on my part, made sure to make physical changes in our house—I changed our bedroom setup so Rohan would have easy access to the bathroom, put in safety rods in the shower along with handles and cleared the furniture to create an easy path for Rohan to practise walking.

Not just Rohan, it would be a change for me and the children too. The therapists impressed upon me how Rohan would be able to mobilise himself. They made him take a shower to give me a real-time feel, and then walked me through the steps of how he would come out of the shower, how he would sit, how he could walk without stumbling. Basically, it was a lesson on the do's and don'ts once Rohan was home.

☙❧

The doctor at the rehab centre set a date for Rohan's discharge: 29 July. I was mentally doing cartwheels but Rohan threw a fit. 'No. I want to leave early.' He refused to listen to any arguments to the contrary.

We compromised on 23 July, provided his recuperation satisfied the doctor. I think that date motivated Rohan to push through all the pain. Every time we spoke after that, he ended our conversations gleefully with, 'Thursday is coming!' The children were getting excited too. They began a countdown of sorts. Every morning, they would ask, 'How many days for Daddy to come home?' I would answer and they would burst into cries of happiness. Kimberly kept them occupied most of the day while I finished off chores and the last touches for Rohan's arrival which included deep cleaning the entire house. Somehow, in the middle of it all, I still could not believe it was happening. It felt real but I did not want to think too far ahead, taking each day at a time.

On the afternoon of 22 July, Bhushan had planned to drive down to Houston and come with me to get Rohan home the next day. We were in the middle of chatting during his drive, when I suddenly had a feeling and blurted out, 'Bhushan, are you bringing Siya?'

Bhushan was astonished. 'I don't believe it! How did you know that?' He was bringing his daughter along as a surprise to us all and while we were conversing on the hands-free, Siya was quiet as a mouse. But once she heard me, she laughingly said, 'Nothing surprises you!'

By evening, we all had butterflies in our stomachs, the good kind. The children were busy blowing up balloons and decorating the house with banners and posters that Kimberly had helped them painstakingly draw and colour over the past week. I beamed on seeing the posters strewn around the living room. Bright colours screaming 'We <3 U Rohan', 'Welcome Superman', 'Welcome Home Rohan'. Some of the crayons were still carelessly lying around, to be used for final touches on the coloured paper the next morning. Bhushan was merry, keeping everyone entertained. The gloom seemed to have lifted, finally.

Rohan called in the evening, in the middle of all the pre-celebrations. But instead of the cheerful note he had been striking all week, his voice was morose. 'I'm feeling uneasy. I can't exercise today.'

It was typical Rohan behaviour; I felt so sure Rohan was feeling lazy to do his exercises and was making up excuses. Surprising for someone who loved sports—both playing and watching—he did not like exercise. But soon, I realised, there was a serious reason behind his reluctance.

☙❧

'I'm feeling much better,' Rohan said over a video-call. His face still looked pale, his eyelids droopy, his cheeks swollen. Contrary to what he said, he looked miserable. It was the evening of 23 July, the day he was to be discharged.

The previous night, the rehab centre had called to say that Rohan was throwing up. He could keep no food or liquids down, and in a few hours, was completely dehydrated. I immediately sensed trouble. 'How could this happen again?' I thought to myself, over and over again, until I wore myself out. The nurse assured me they were going to take Rohan to get x-rays done and start an intravenous drip.

I tossed and turned all night, my stomach gurgling. This time, I plunged into the dark abyss of despair. Somewhere, deep down, I had lost hope. There was no chance Rohan was coming home as planned. When Vivaan came to my bed, snuggled up next to me, and asked, 'When is Daddy coming?' I had no answer for him. His crushed face broke me, almost.

We were so close to victory. So close.

The next call from the hospital escalated our fears. A CT scan found Rohan's gall bladder was inflamed. It was just 10 in the morning when he was put on antibiotics. Bhushan and I sat at the breakfast nook, worry written on our faces. Neither of us could eat anything, we just drank coffee to calm our nerves. The children sensed the negative energy but Siya, the oldest among them, tried to play with the rest to keep their minds at ease. 'Come, let's finish the posters,' she said, leading the trio away.

'What next?' I asked. 'We will need to observe your husband. If his condition does not improve after two or three days with the antibiotics, we would have to move him to a hospital to operate.'

Bhushan and I cried out together. The light at the end of the tunnel had suddenly disappeared. I appealed to Sai Baba in my mind. It was a Thursday. After getting Baba's darshan, how could this happen on his divine day? My mind just could not comprehend anything for a few minutes as I stared ahead, my hands gripping the coffee cup tight until my knuckles were white. The silence was deafening. We could only wait at that point. Bhushan kept the families informed, I just could not talk to anyone. I needed space to breathe and calm down.

It must have been a miracle but after the first round of antibiotics, Rohan was better. The staff called to give an update before Rohan did. He had managed to keep down some apple juice by the end of the day. I could see him forcefully sipping the tetra-pack juice; trying hard not to cry. My heart went out to him. Instead of being home with his family, he was still in a sterile room staring at the white walls.

The following day was critical; would Rohan feel better or would his condition worsen? I'm not the gambling kind but I felt I had won the jackpot because Rohan was better when I got the call from the rehab centre. The gall bladder operation seemed unlikely because the antibiotics were lessening the inflammation. However, a side report did state Rohan's liver could function better. A liquid diet of water and apple juice, with a bit of lumpy jelly thrown in the mix, seemed to do the trick. I could almost hear a smile in his voice during the evening call.

Rohan could eat light food on 25 July. Toast and crackers were consumed with ease, washed down with apple juice. 'I'm feeling much better, don't worry,' he told me in the morning.

I was speaking with Bhushan in the afternoon when the rehab centre called. They uttered the magic words that immediately uplifted our moods. Rohan was ready to be discharged the very next day!

Bhushan whooped with joy. He had gone back to Austin and immediately decided to drive down again with Siya. 'There is no way I won't be there when Rohan comes home,' he stated.

The air at home was filled with excitement. The children had gotten their hopes up high. The twins had made another poster with Jessica's help, while Vivaan was diligently cleaning a soccer ball. He understood Rohan could not play but he wanted to show it to him nevertheless. It was their thing, this soccer madness.

I was emotionally drained. My mind could not comprehend that it was over. The hell into which we had descended over the last four months was finally giving way to heaven. Bhushan and the parents rejoiced over a group call, while I was fearful about showing too much excitement. I was haunted by the thought that things might not work out again. I couldn't eat a thing, instead cooked a few of Rohan's favourite things once again like I had a few days ago. When Rohan called that night, all the children wanted to talk to him. They were screaming with joy and I could see Rohan beaming in bed. His body was still sore from the vomiting. 'Tomorrow...' he promised, blowing the children air kisses.

Bhushan gave me a bear hug before we all went to bed early, in preparation for 26 July. 'You did it, Manasi,' he said, squeezing my shoulders. 'He is coming home.'

I turned away, mumbling something. I did not dare hope until I'd actually see him cross the threshold. Over the last four months, I had been mentally prepared for Rohan to return in any shape. I couldn't imagine life without him. And finally, it seemed, it was all coming true. The momentous occasion was just some hours away.

PART THREE

ROHAN'S STORY

Homecoming

I didn't know where I was. My mind registered white walls just beyond, but what did it mean? I felt exhausted, my eyelids drooping, too tired to tilt my head. I was breathing but couldn't move. I could see tubes everywhere from the corners of my eyes. I could hear the echo of breathing around me. Was it my breath, and was I breathing that loud? The sound was calming, at first, a steady rise and fall but it soon turned to fear. I was suddenly terrified. If I could, I would have started to panic, but I did not have the energy. In a moment, everything faded away…

I heard my name in the realms of my subconscious. 'Who's that?' I wondered. I could see myself standing tall, wearing the old grey sweats Manasi hates with all her heart, looking around the dark space. I could hear someone calling me, but there was no one. And there was darkness, once again.

My head felt heavy, my body felt drugged but a face came into view. It was a face I did not know. She was saying something, I could see her mouth moving slowly, but I could not grasp the words. Everything felt abuzz, I looked down at the inner part of my elbow; there were tubes connected, covered by white tape. And I thought of needles. 'Who did this to me?' I wondered again, before my eyes shut.

The next time I woke up, I thought of Manasi. I was not groggy, my mind felt clear, fresh after a long nap. I thought of her face, her smile. But I could not move, my body felt sore and battered. The white walls seemed to have closed in but, wait, what was that? I saw pieces of paper and what was that picture? My eyes took a while to focus but yes, it was…us. The children, Manasi and I. But, why was there a picture of us on the wall? Where was I? Why did my mouth feel so dry? I was parched, I needed to drink something.

I saw a nurse hovering around me, her back turned. I tried to call out to her, get her attention. She suddenly turned with a huge smile, 'I see a bit of grimace! And I see movement in your arm! You will be fine,' she tried to assure me. I had no idea what she was referring to. Then, suddenly she thrust a phone in front of my face—and I saw Manasi. She looked tired. Her face seemed taut, she had dark circles under her eyes. Was she alright? What had happened to her? I wanted to speak to her but as I tried, I realised the futility because I could feel a tube in my throat. I almost gagged, I wanted to take the tube out, rip it out so I could talk. But I had no strength left to do the deed. I suddenly felt spent, sapped of all energy. And I dozed off, no recollection for how long.

I felt I was afloat, somewhere in the clouds, light as a feather. I think I saw a ray of light shooting towards me from afar; the ray slowly enveloped me and then, I felt it penetrate my body. It did not feel awkward, something about it was soothing. I felt at peace, my soul felt nourished. And I slept like a baby.

I don't know how long I hovered in the realms of the two worlds, sometimes in the conscious, and then, visiting the unconscious. But slowly, I could feel my body telling me to wake up. I was hit with a sudden heaviness. The insides of my head felt clouded. It felt something was inside, shaking my brains from the inside. I understood I was lying in a hospital bed but I didn't know how long I had been there. I could hear Manasi's voice on the phone, yet I could not lift my arms high enough to reach out to her. But she looked happy when I creased my cheeks to form a smile. I could understand her, it was taking time. The nurses were everywhere, so attentive, so eager to help.

Though I felt safe, I could also feel my body waging an inner battle. I felt my insides curdling, yet because of the tube attached to my throat, I could barely speak. A rasped croak is best to describe the sound my voice was making. I made out a nurse saying I was running a fever, but I did not know why. I felt fine internally, in between bouts of heaviness.

Suddenly, one day, there was Manasi. In the flesh. I thought I was dreaming, but no, there she was. Her eyes were welling up as she held my hand. I wanted to tell her so many things but couldn't. So we stayed silent, looking at each other, hand in hand. A calmness had descended upon us; I wished I could stay like that forever.

⚬⚬⚬

'Hell', I thought and groaned, trying to move my useless body. My lower back was itching, but I could not reach behind to relieve the sensation. It was exasperating not being able to do simple tasks, tasks we take for granted.

I felt frustrated. My body strength was returning but the whole recovery process felt so long-winded. I was less delirious and returning to the coronavirus-affected world. I knew the world was in tatters because I could hear the hospital staff discuss it, even though I found it difficult to speak. I tried using an alphabet board, but soon, lost all patience to type out everything I wanted to say.

I needed to be able to speak.

What if I was never able to? The thought was terrifying. Not even watching a horror film had ever jolted me like the thought. The tube was a constant source of discomfort and I wanted to tear it away. I was frightened:

What if it became a part of me? The second thought that kept bothering me was what if I could never walk again? How would I live my life? I lay in bed but despair flooded me. There was no escape. I still could not get up on my own, nor did I have the strength in my legs to walk. I felt hopelessness engulf me, and I had nowhere to hide.

My aversion to needles is thanks to my long personal history of hospital visits. I know I'm accident-prone but my brain could not comprehend the severity of the situation this time. I knew this hospital visit felt different to all the others but I did not understand why, until much later. It is also the longest I ever stayed at a hospital. And it was driving me crazy the number of times the nurses would come and draw blood. I'm sure they had done it during the days I lay unconscious in bed but now that I had regained some of my senses, every prick was excruciatingly painful. One prick, thrice a day, left me screaming in my mind, croaking physically. I was later told the staff was unable to find any other veins, leaving my thumb and index finger open to needles. One day, I wondered in despair if getting out of the hospital was even a reality. I had reached a state of anguish I did not know I possessed.

I recollected the group video-call the day Manasi had come to visit. I saw my parents, Manasi's parents, Bhushan and Priya; they were all egging me on to get better. I saw their faces, frightened and finally, relieved but still tearful. Everyone was crying, I still did not understand why. Slowly, comprehension dawned: what they were seeing was a mirror image of what I was feeling. They had been scared for me as I lay there semi-conscious, I was now scared for myself after regaining consciousness.

I was moved to the PCU soon after Manasi's visit. At first, I thought of it excitedly, a new room, a new place; but, as the hours went by, my restlessness grew. I knew something was not right, I just didn't know what triggered it. What helped in the dark bout was seeing Manasi every single day. She could come visit me in my new windowless room (she told me later there was a window but I was too mentally anguished to take note at that point); I felt suffocated, breathless but just seeing her daily for the stipulated time kept me going.

Unlike the ICU, my new abode felt restrictive despite the name 'progressive'. I felt uneasy throughout the day, I felt no one was paying any attention to me. There was no one to communicate with even though I was still rasping. I'm not much of a talker, I prefer to listen. But at that moment, if I could, I would talk with anyone about anything under the sun. I think the first time it really hit me that I was not going home any time soon was when it took me over 15 minutes, with help, to get from the bed to a chair. A physical therapist had come, and in between the tests, tried to limber my limbs. He would make me sit by the side of the bed, which hurt until I got used to it. The day he helped me up for the first time, my legs felt like jelly, I could have been knocked over by the wind. He kept pushing me when I wanted to give up. 'Just a little more, just a little more,' he kept repeating till

I wanted to scream at him. When I sat down, the initial moment shocked me. I was completely out of breath, desperately trying to gulp more air. And then, fear set in. If just getting to a chair left me winded, how on earth would I be able to walk?

Day turned to night, night turned to day; I could not keep track of time. I was lonely, my anxiety skyrocketing, feeling as if my heart would jump out of my chest beating loudly. My dreams were overwhelmingly strange. When Manasi came to visit daily, I would try and tell her; communicate with hand gestures and whatever words I could formulate. I told her I was playing cricket with Kapil and Vivaan. I remember I was batting to the former India captain's bowling. I may have even scored a six. That part is blurry but I do distinctly recall Kapil's face, coming at me with lightning speed, as Vivaan cheered me in the background.

One night, I dreamt of an island. A virgin sandy white beach, coconut palms jutting out from the middle of the island, the tiny strip of land surrounded by the deep blue sea. I had always wanted to go to the Maldives, to take a seaplane ride from one atoll to the next. Maybe I was there? I wanted to jump and do cartwheels, but was happy to take in the breeze and lie on the sand. I felt at peace without the tubes and wires sticking out of me.

'Vasanti was mentioning you had gone to a happy place,' Manasi explained. She had earlier told me about the affirmations, printed and stuck by the edge of the bed. I wanted to believe everything Manasi was telling me but somewhere at the back of my mind my anxiety was clouding my judgement. Maybe that's why another night I dreamt I had gotten up from the hospital bed and left the dreary place but reluctantly came back and got under the covers. I really did want to leave, you see.

My stay at the PCU was also restrictive. I could not press the call button by the bed for nurses because I had been admonished many times. I wanted some comfort but instead, I think, I really think, my hands were tied at some point. My mind is hazy on the details. I felt as if I was being manhandled as the nurses changed me. It was rough, too rough as I remember it. I sometimes lost control of my bowels and could not do anything about it. Was the force necessary? Or was I hallucinating all of it because I was so depressed? I wanted Manasi by my side constantly. She would calm me down during her visits, try to tell me I would soon be moved to something called LTACH. After a point I didn't care, refusing to listen to whatever she wanted to convey. I just wanted, desperately, to get out of the PCU. However, in all the darkness, I did find support in the form of my respiratory therapist, Sally.[1] She tirelessly worked to help me on her shifts, pushed me to do better so I could go home sooner.

Vasanti had mentioned to Manasi that a prolonged stay in this place would hamper my recovery. Maybe

---

1   *Name changed to protect the privacy of the individual*

I could feel her healing touch in my soul because the warning signs that the PCU was not my cup of tea was prevalent. I was growing more miserable by the day despite staff saying I was doing better medically. One day, I got so anxious that I tried to run out. Attempted to. I thought I had jumped out of bed, in reality I tried to slide out of it and fell. My legs buckled, as there was no strength in the calves which I had developed over years of playing so much sport. I cried out, not in pain but in embarrassment. Two nurses came rushing to my aid, then tucked me away like a naughty child. It was that night that my oxygen levels dropped dramatically. The failed getaway was damaging for my internal organs, because everything in my body was still fragile. If only I had not done what I did, maybe I could have moved to the LTACH sooner, cutting my stay at the PCU short.

Manasi's face fell when she saw me one evening at the PCU. 'What happened?' she asked, concerned.

'COVID test...mess,' I said, slowly, trying to enunciate each word. A new fear had crept up that morning when a routine nasal swab drew blood. Manasi had propped up my hopes of leaving this place soon but when the nurse inserted the cotton swab up my nose, it left me convulsed in pain. I felt she was jabbing the elongated bud into my brain matter, causing me to wail in anguish. I could feel the jab was bungled because a tiny trail of blood left my nose, dropping onto the nursing gown. The crimson colour was jarring against the pristine whiteness. I had to test negative twice in order to move on from this hell.

No one really told me anything unless I croaked to get their attention. I was asleep when suddenly I felt my bed move. I opened my eyes in shock; sure enough, four nurses were moving my bed. My heart dropped, I knew this had to do with *that* test, I knew it. 'What… happened?' I questioned to no one in particular. Either they didn't hear me, or they were deliberately ignoring me. But I was no quitter, my parents did not raise me to be one.

'What…happened?' I asked again, this time with more forceful hoarseness.

It worked. One of the nurses looked at me and confirmed my nightmare. 'You have tested positive. We need to isolate you.'

I felt afraid as I was being wheeled away but then, anger coursed through my veins. I could visualise Manasi's anguished face in front of me, I knew how upset she would be hearing the negative news. I fought off angry tears; I wanted to see my children so badly. I was missing their warmth, their smiles. At that point, I felt the world around me had crashed, and all that was left was darkened despair. My body went limp, my mind numb.

⊗⊗

I thought about the time I went to Flushing Meadows on a whim. It was late summer, the 2010 USA Open was on in full swing. I had come from Houston to New York for just a day. I wrapped up the meeting and, on a whim, caught a train to Queens. Wearing a formal suit and tie, I cheered on Robin Söderling as he easily defeated American Taylor Dent. Söderling had had a fantastic year—the final at Roland Garros, the narrow loss to Federer in the fourth round at Wimbledon where he was only broken once, a jump in ATP ranking points… watching the Swede play was a lesson in mastery.

Exhilarated, I then saw Sania Mirza playing a singles match. Shoaib Malik was in the crowd, cheering his wife on. The Pakistani cricketer's marriage to India's beloved tennis player earlier in the year had shocked the sporting world, not to mention the public of the two countries. I watched as Sania's magnificent forehand ripped apart her opponent, drawing applause from the stands. As a final forehand winner gave Sania the match, I quickly made my way to Shoaib's box. He obliged me with a picture, and I wished I could have taken a photo with Sania too. Unfortunately, I had over-extended my stay: if I lingered any longer, I would miss my company flight back.

'Why are you laughing?' Manasi asked, surprised to hear me chuckle. We were waiting inside the LTACH facility before I could be taken to my room. I was tired, almost dozing but I kept recalling Manasi's face when I told her of my USA Open adventure that night, almost a decade ago. She had been angry, wanting me to fly her to New York so she, too, could see the matches!

The consequent COVID tests came back negative, allowing the move to LTACH. I was so relieved that I did not have to go back into the PCU. Just thinking about the place made me break out in a sweat. Manasi and I had just taken an ambulance ride together. Going inside one did not seem scary after the March ordeal. I knew why I remained calm: because Manasi was with me. How I had missed her when she was not allowed to visit after the mismanaged positive test.

I must have dozed off sometime during the paperwork for admission because when I woke up, it was early morning. I saw a line drawn by sunlight known as raxeira across my bed. I breathed out, my heart felt lighter just knowing I could look out of a window from my bed. The world did not seem gloomy any longer.

That was the day I truly realised the extent of my damaged body. And it was a rude awakening. It boggled my mind how one sneeze could change my life. The doctor who was to look after my recovery asked, 'Do you know what has happened to you?' Seeing me shake my head, he explained without scaring me, how much effort I had to put in to get back some semblance of normalcy. 'The task will not be easy, but you have to put in all the effort you can muster. Things will progress. It is all about the baby steps.'

When I first remembered that godawful sneeze, I felt angry. I wanted to break every bone in that person's body. But I had to let that feeling dissipate. I *had* to look ahead. If I wanted to go home, I would have to be able to live without help. And once I set my mind to that, I got to work. Recurring irritations and annoyances aside, I wanted to see my children. When Manasi had shown me a video with the three of them longingly call out to me, I wanted to rush home. I wanted to bear hug them. 'Fight Rohan, fight,' I told myself when my body refused to cooperate during physical therapy. I needed to get better for them.

In the beginning, just stretching my arms above my head felt like a tall task. But, when the therapist made me sit on a chair, I felt I would collapse with exhaustion. I cannot begin to describe the pain I felt from the neck down. I thought my body would not be able to bear the weight and crumble into a messy heap. The chair torture would last for an hour. When you want time to pass, it invariably goes slowly. Just twenty minutes in, I would call the therapist to take me to bed. 'You still have forty more minutes, Rohan,' she would scold.

I would complain to Manasi every single day, 'They tortured me.' She would laugh and hold my hand. I could see the dark circles under her eyes slowly fading. Just the thought that she was better brought me joy.

Over the next week, I was able to get up from bed and stand without support. The first time, using a walker, I managed to go up to the door of my room and back. A mere nine or so steps, but I felt I had conquered Mount Everest. As I pushed to walk more, my mind went back to the twins' baby years. When they were learning to walk, we would encourage them to stumble after they had just taken a few steps. A fall made them try harder to get up, try again. I was going through the same process, albeit some decades older.

The leg presses were killing me. I thought I had strong calves but a look at them now made me whimper. Where had all those muscles gone? Jerry,[2] my nurse, would encourage me to do a bit more. One day when Manasi was there, Jerry made me do a set in front of her. I was sweating buckets, but managed to get through the count. 'Put…me in…bed,' I struggled to say. Jerry looked at me, then at Manasi who was watching me intently, and said scornfully, 'C'mon man, even my eight-year-old can do more.' That taunt sparked a fire: I pushed myself harder to prove him wrong.

Manasi had dropped off a phone which only had her number and that of close family members. At last, I felt connected with her after god knows how many weeks apart. I shook the pain of the PCU off my mind; at least here I could text instead of lying in bed all alone listening to the news. And I did not want to hear what was going on outside the LTACH walls—the deaths across the world, the rising number of confirmed cases, every country struggling, clinical trials, the shocking death of George Floyd. It was depressing, filling my mind with despair. Instead, I would smile looking at Manasi's texts, slowly re-reading all of them; watching videos of the children; and reply to messages to help the dexterity in my fingers improve. I would text Manasi each day the number of

---

2   *Name changed to protect the privacy of the individual*

steps I took. The day I wrote '92 feet', Manasi whooped with joy. I myself could not believe it!

One thing that annoyed me was the neurologist's daily visit. Every morning he would put two fingers in front of my face and ask, 'How many do you see?'

Did the man think me mad? Of course, I could see two fingers. I saw those damned two fingers every day. One morning, I lost my cool and stammered, 'Why are…you…doing this?'

His reply shocked me. 'We found you suffered a stroke. It could have happened due to the cardiac arrest.'

'Wha…what do you mean?' I stuttered.

'You were very lucky, young man. You coded twice.'

My head went into a tailspin. I had no idea about that. I could have died. Somehow I calmed my nerves, and when Manasi came to visit that evening, I could not share what I had learnt. It was too soon, too scary. Manasi obviously knew and I understood she did not want me to know. I did not want her to worry, she already had a lot on her plate. So I tried not to show my nervousness, and instead, launched into discussions about food. I love food, our whole family loves to eat. Only recently, I had begun to eat semi-solid foods after the doctors made me do a swallow test. Manasi had begun to send home-made dishes, dal and rice or well-boiled pasta so it melted in my mouth. It was a relief to be able to eat again. Just some bites were more than enough to make me feel I was growing stronger.

During one of my speech therapy sessions, a doctor casually mentioned that I would be 'getting out of here' next week. If I could have, I would have danced all night. The words felt like music to my ears. I was mentally cartwheeling and shaking my hips to my 1980s jam when Manasi brought me crashing down to earth. 'You are going to a rehab centre, not home.'

Whatever did she mean? Of course I was going home. That is what the doctor had said. I was fine, I did not need further rehab. Why was she dampening my euphoria?

I was getting cross no matter how much Manasi tried to explain things. I would not hear any of it. At that moment, I felt my hopes dash, everything was back to square one. If I was not getting better, did it mean the tube would forever be stuck with me? I could have cried, I wanted to go home. I needed to go home. And she was denying me the opportunity to do so.

൭൫

'How are you feeling, *beta*?'

I could see the concern on my mother's face. 'Fine, better.'

'Did you eat yet?'

'Pasta *khaya* (ate). Manasi *ne laya tha* (brought it).'

She broke into a smile. 'You will soon go home. You just have to get more fit. We are visiting a temple every day to pray for you.'

I smiled and raised my arm to wave but it fell on the bed. The day's therapy had left me exhausted. My eyelids fluttered, unable to stay open. My head drooped, and I heard my mother saying 'Bye' from far away.

It had been a few days since I heard about the rehab centre. I was still angry, but it was actually the neurologist who had knocked some sense in me. 'Rohan, what would happen if a plane crashed in a rural area? Less casualties, right? Now, what if the plane crashed in a busy metropolis? The casualties would skyrocket, wouldn't they? Your stroke probably occurred in a part of your brain where sensory functions are not used much. If it had happened in a vital area, Rohan, you would not even be able to talk to me. Just think of this time as a way to improve yourself. You are still weak, though you may not comprehend that. You'd rather be independent than be dependent on your family, right?'

He was right. Oh, it was so infuriating. I had to have some semblance of independence at home. Right now, I was not even close.

When I was moved to the rehab centre, Manasi rode with me holding my hand in the back of the ambulance. It was evening, I think, when I was brought down to the waiting ambulance. I saw the sky and breathed in fresh air. It felt good; I can never take looking at a sky for granted again. It was also the twins' birthday and I wished I was with them. I wanted to see their faces when they cut the cake. I thought about the last birthday, when Aria had gotten frosting on her nose and Ayaan had come too close to the lit candles. They were a pair of lovable clowns. 'I will cut a cake with you two soon,' I promised myself, squeezing Manasi's hand tighter as the ambulance wailed, taking us to our destination.

When the therapists at the centre asked me my goals, I looked at them quizzically. It was the day after I was admitted. I had not slept properly. I was still tired from shifting from one room to another, being awoken in the middle of the night for a COVID test, and annoyed that a nurse drew blood from my right index finger because she could find no other vein. But, in spite of all the negativity, there was a ray of hope.

I was feeling that way because the dratted tube was taken out just before the ambulance ride. I remembered fretting at the hospital, trying to gesture to a nurse how I would never be able to speak again despite her assurances that I would get my voice back. I recalled my despair. I had never believed the day would come when I could speak without the tube jutting out. But today, there was no tube. I felt a lightness in my heart, a feeling of comfort that one day this ordeal would be over. It was all a matter of time.

The therapist again repeated himself. 'What are your goals?'

'I want to go home.' I was able to say the entire sentence without a pause. Then, I explained what I had in mind. 'I need to be able to walk into my home.'

'Well, and that is what we will prepare you for,' the therapist replied, smiling.

The focus at the rehab centre was on physical and mental therapy. I eventually got used to the workload, the urgency to get home playing a huge motivational role. Manasi's messages were also a morale booster. Even if I felt tired, I asked for more exercises. On most days, dog-tired after the workouts, I would quickly eat dinner by 6 pm and then doze off with the television still on.

I had been away long enough. Manasi realised my determination on family training days when she came over to understand how things would be once I was home. I began to re-learn the basics—how to brush my teeth, how to use the washroom getting up from a wheelchair without help, how to be able to shower and then dry myself. The focus was not on regaining upper and lower body strength but conditioning the body to do daily activities around the house. I was often taken to a mock kitchen area and asked to get up from the wheelchair to perform mundane exercises. They would range from walking to the refrigerator and opening the door to closing cabinets. The real pain came when I had to bend and put a cup, in which I had make-belief coffee, in the dishwasher. Simple, routine stuff that knocked the wind out of me. Despite the pain, the positivity kept me going. Completing the tasks felt like a win, nearer to the end-goal of regaining my independence.

To get my mind sharper and be able to get back to work eventually, I was taken to a computer room and made to type on a keyboard. 'Browse the web,' they said. Due to texting, my dexterity was better but I was still slow. At times when I got frustrated, the therapists would let me be. 'It'll happen, you'll see,' they encouraged. One day, they made me dance to Michael Jackson. I could not do the moon walk but could happily tap my feet standing up for an extended period. I played table tennis as a child and really enjoy watching one of the world's fastest sports on television. One day the therapists made me pick up a table tennis bat and hit a few rallies against an opponent. It was annoying not to hit the ball with finesse but I had to remind myself they were gauging my reflexes and hand-eye coordination, not my stance or ability to play the sport! I was often taken to the courtyard in a wheelchair, given headphones playing my favourite music, and told to get up and walk. I guess the music beats made me want to dance, and I had to get up in order to do so.

'Wow, I can easily stand without help,' I suddenly realised in the middle of a therapy session one morning at the gym. I was overwhelmed with emotion; just some weeks ago I had thought I would never be able to walk again. I had already progressed from an automatic wheelchair to a manual one, and now used a walker on most occasions. I sniffed away the tears that were threatening to gush out. 'No, move, Rohan,' I said to myself as Prince's 'Raspberry beret' played in my ears.

'You've made excellent progress, Rohan,' an administrator said to Manasi and me during a family training meet. 'We can release you by the end of the month.'

'No.'

Manasi looked at me in surprise. 'I want to leave early.' I refused to budge from my decision. Some back and forth later, the centre agreed to release me on 23 July, provided the therapists were happy with my progress.

Now that a deadline had been set, I pushed myself to take on more exercise sets. I was doing more leg presses, more walkarounds, more vocal training, even trying to shoot a basketball in the gym to gain strength. I was doing everything and more to be able to go home and live normally. Sometimes, I was asked to slow down, but shook my head and pushed on. The thought of reuniting with my children drove me.

Despite all my efforts, there could be a potential barrier that could ruin all my hard work. I would have to pass an evaluation before I could be discharged. The evaluation would determine if I would need any equipment at home. All the weeks of preparation would ultimately boil down to a six-minute walk test that would appraise how my body, especially the respiratory system, was handling stress. Failure to meet an acceptable mark meant I would have to use an oxygen cylinder at home. I really, really did not want that.

I was nervous—I would be lying if I said I wasn't—on the day of the exam. I kept telling myself to stay calm and carry on, the meme playing over and over in my head. I tried not to put too much pressure on myself. Six minutes of walking later, I felt great; and to my surprise, realised I passed the stress test with ease! My oxygen level did not drop below 92 (oxygen saturation of 95-100 per cent is normal in healthy adults) which satisfied the therapists. I was elated the whole day, until I dozed off in the evening with a smile plastered on my face.

ॐ

'I can't do it.'

I sank into the wheelchair, feeling sick. I was at the laundry room with an occupational therapist. She was instructing me to put clothes in the washer, like I would at home. My body was not cooperating.

'Go on, I know you can,' she insisted.

I mustered all the strength I had to chuck the sheet inside. 'Can you push me back, please?' I whispered. I had no strength to turn the wheels. It was 22 July, the day before I was to be discharged, a day I had been dreaming of since I woke up. By evening, my stomach was hurting and I needed medication to fall asleep. However, nothing alleviated the pain. Instead, the cramps got worse and left me literally sobbing into my pillow. The resident prescribed more medication and called for the doctor. I threw up everything I had ingested just before he came. The nurse on duty tried to give me some apple juice because I was dehydrated by then. But I threw that up as well. I just could not keep anything down.

'Antibiotics, please,' I begged the doctor. 'Not without running tests,' he said. Though I had tears streaming down my cheeks, he would not budge. When the results finally came in, they determined what I knew all along—I had an infection. My heart had sunk by then, I knew I would not be discharged just yet.

The doctors scared Manasi, suggesting a possibility of gallstones. But they ultimately found nothing. It was a silly infection that decided to act up at a crucial time. Over the next two days, I got better and the pain disappeared with medication. I could eat some fruits and cheese and keep down more apple juice. Finally, after many more tests, the doctors at the facility deemed I could be discharged on 26 July. I could not wait. I could finally hold my children in my arms. It felt like I was waking up from a dream.

When my phone pinged on Sunday morning, I had been awake for hours with excitement. It was Manasi.

'Good morning. I can't wait to have you home!'

Manasi had mentioned that my parents had gone to the Ganesh temple to pray the day before in Mumbai. Manasi's parents, along with Bhushan, Priya and Manasi had participated in a prayer meeting for my well-being late Saturday night. It touched me—as it is, I could not quantify the amount of prayers and blessings I had received from everywhere—family, friends, colleagues, strangers. At that moment, I felt I was the luckiest chap in the world. I was abreast of news of the pandemic around the world—heads of states testing positive, confirmed case counts increasing, death tolls breaking all previous records. So many had not survived this damned virus, and yet, I did. I fought to survive, Manasi fought to keep me alive. And I was fortunate enough to finally go home, having won the war.

My bags were packed, I was dressed in my favourite T-shirt and shorts, wearing the most comfortable bright yellow socks. I could not stop smiling. Manasi entered the room and I could see her eyes sparkle with happiness.

I lost track of time when we hugged, neither wanting to let go. We could not believe this day had finally arrived. We had hoped and prayed, but this was reality. She walked beside my wheelchair as two nurses wheeled me outside to the waiting car. We kept glancing at each other in excitement. Yet, there was a slight sense of nervousness too because it was finally happening. Who knew a sneeze could put me inside hospital walls for four months?

Bhushan was waiting outside and whipped out his phone as we came out the doors. He was doing a group call—the parents, the children, Priya. Everyone was clapping, both sets of parents were tearing up with joy. Even the nurses joined in! I was ecstatic, the applause felt thunderous. I felt I was on top of the world. Bhushan kept saying, 'You did it, you did it' as I got up from the wheelchair and walked to the car seat, pumping my arms into the air like a batsman who had just scored a ton to save India on the pitch. I had scored a win because I was walking out of the medical facility alive and well. I was going home to my loved ones, beating all odds.

The happiness in the car was exhilarating. And to my surprise, as our home came into view, I saw Vivaan, Ayaan, Aria and Siya standing with posters and balloons on the sidewalk, each screaming with joy and waving so hard I thought they would dislocate joints! 'Superman', 'We <3 u'—I held back tears reading the words on the colourful posters they had painted. I could not wait to squish each of them and slobber them with kisses.

Manasi conducted a small prayer before I finally

crossed the threshold into our home. It's an ancient prayer learnt from our elders in which salt and mustard seeds are used to remove the ill effects of the evil eye. As she finished the mantra, she looked into my eyes. I felt happiness wash over me; a sense of calm descended on us both, drowning out all tertiary noise. We held each other's hands and walked in together.

I looked around the living room, taking it all in. The children ran inside and surrounded me, wrapping their arms around my legs and waist. I hugged them back, laughing because I was not dreaming the moment.

I finally let out a long sigh of relief. A deep breath. I could not yet believe that I was home, and I had no intentions of leaving for a long, long time.

Epilogue: Stepping up the pace

26 July 2021

I suddenly awoke, my heart beating wildly against my chest. Sweat had soaked my pillow, the grey night-time tee clinging to me. Beads of sweat rolled down my forehead as I tried to wipe them away without waking Manasi. It was dark outside, everything around me was silent. I could hear crickets outside the window, breaking the still of the night. Manasi turned beside me, and I saw her face light up, a stream of moonlight shining on her face. I couldn't believe that a year had passed. My hand involuntarily touched my throat, touching the scar lines that would take a long time to fade. Maybe they never would.

Today marks my one-year anniversary of returning home alive. To have made it despite the odds and slim chances; in a world still filled with terror by an unseen evil, a virus so deadly that it keeps evolving and creating new strains to create pandemonium.

I looked at my toes and wiggled them intentionally. Something so silly, yet a little over a year back I thought I would never be able to do this again. I have always looked ahead in my life, yet I can't help but sometimes relive the time I felt I never would have been able to talk or walk. It had been terrifying. I remember the pain, excruciating needle pricks that drove me mad. The tightly clenched fists to keep myself from crying out hoarsely. At one point, I remember lying in the hospital bed with silent tears streaming down my face. On a night like this, I would become a burden, I had thought. But I was wrong. There *was* a light at the end of the tunnel.

I can recollect the parade like it was yesterday. It was just some days after Manasi and Bhushan drove me home, the target we all had worked hard towards since I came to my senses. Manasi had put up a chair on the porch outside our home, and I gingerly walked towards it. I didn't know what to expect but as soon as I saw a line of cars slowly coming towards our house, I broke into a smile. Our friends and neighbours had decided to show their support via a drive-through parade. I remember being overwhelmed because so many friendly faces stopped by. They didn't physically come up and hug me; as I sat on a chair, slightly tired from the exertion,

I felt loved. I remember the gratitude in Manasi's eyes throughout the day. It had been hell for her to manage everything on her own in such trying times. I am blessed to have such a wife. I knew how special she was on our first date, and I am so glad she said yes to spending her life with me.

My children were so excited to have their father back. The initial months of the pandemic had been hard for them. I didn't mind one bit that during my first week at home, they would come and give me random hugs. They would unexpectedly barge into my room as I did my exercises to say, 'I love you, Daddy.' I felt treasured.

I knew I had a mountain to climb; coming home was only a small step in the greater scheme of things. Now, it was trying to get back to how I was before I fell ill. I knew Manasi was worried. She was trying hard to put on a brave face but at the hospital, or later in the LTACH, I was always near medical professionals. Now, it was just us trying to reach goals we had set for ourselves with medical inputs. It happened so many times that I would wake up to see her face hovering over me, watching me intently. She was looking out for skipped heartbeats. Though my initial thought would be of irritation, I would quickly tell myself to let go of the negativity; it was a tough adjustment for both and we didn't need anything to upset the flow.

My emotions would fluctuate. Sometimes, I would feel guilty. When Vivi asked me if we could play soccer together, I felt angry, and then immediately afterwards, heartbroken. I was angry because I put my family through the trauma of those months when I hovered between life and death, and now that I was back, I was still in a shell which would take a long time to break. I took my eight-year-old's hands, and looked into his eyes. 'I will kick a ball with you by Christmas,' I solemnly promised him.

I tried hard to rest and relax, not over-exert. It was difficult. At times, I wanted to speed up the process in an attempt to fix myself faster. I am no professional athlete, even though I used to be fit. I started by trying to be independent—to wean myself off the walker (which I accomplished in a little over a month), walk up the stairs (another tick-off around the same time), shower and brush my teeth without help, focus on breathing exercises to increase my lung capacity and not let my oxygen level drop below 90 (my breathlessness slowly began to dissipate), and phase myself back to work after copious sessions of occupational therapy at the LTACH. A friend of Manasi's, a physiotherapist by profession, was of great help around this time, aiding in improving my mobility and overall strength, especially my legs.

It was sometime in August, a month after I had returned, that I went for my first drive. When I stayed away from my family in Virginia, drives in the evening after work would often help me when I missed them. I would drive aimlessly to try and discover new places, mentally taking notes where I would bring Manasi and the children when they visited me. The moment I got behind the wheel, something stirred in me. I felt muscle memory rushing back, and at that moment, I knew I was on the right track. That I was definitely getting better. 'Get out now,' Manasi laughed, 'once around the neighbourhood is enough for now.' I smiled and caught her hand. I was soon able to drive to the physiotherapy sessions on my own, which came as a big morale booster.

My colleagues had been extremely supportive throughout the process, and I wanted to get back to work. However, first, I had to go for a check-up. Coronavirus was still raging in September—it had become the third leading cause of death in the country. To make matters worse, a case had recently been reported of re-infection which was more severe the second time. As if that wasn't enough, Phase 3 trials of three vaccines were taking place around the world but there was news of one of them being halted as a 'routine action'. Apparently, a patient in the United Kingdom's arm of the trial had an adverse reaction. Manasi tried to remain hopeful through all this, but I knew she had been affected by the news. I was too. The world needed a vaccine because the high numbers were still alarming.

Meeting Dr Sheth, albeit virtually, was not the best 'first check-up'. We discussed my continuing arrhythmia. 'I'll send you a heart monitor to keep check,' he said. The risk of untreated arrhythmia is a risk of a cardiac arrest. I did not want a repeat of the fateful day when I coded twice. Manasi still has nightmares of the day I truly hit rock bottom. I was prescribed medication. My heartbeats were monitored for almost a month while we went to the pulmonologist. The walk test showed my lung capacity at 33 per cent. Not great news, to be honest. It felt frustrating but I did not want to relapse to how I felt stuck in the hospital bed. I kept telling myself that I was getting better. I was weak still, but not in the condition I was three-four months ago. Going back to work helped at this time, for it kept my mind occupied. My colleagues welcomed me virtually with open arms, easing me back on projects. 'Don't rush back,' they insisted from Virginia.

The joy of meeting Dr Sheth in person, to be able to thank him for all his efforts in October was marred by terrible news. I could feel Manasi's body go tense, her fists clench under the table. Disappointment was writ large on my face; I felt the rug being pulled from under my feet. 'Rohan, frankly, we don't know what to expect. Or what will happen or can happen. You are a guinea pig, we have never had a patient like you before,' the doctor said. He tried to be kind, but we went numb trying to understand the implications of his words. My Ejection Fraction (EF) was at 25-30 per cent. Any reading below 35 per cent qualifies for a pacemaker. I was prescribed blood pressure medication in addition to the preventive heart failure medicines from last month. Dr Sheth really was not happy with the condition of my heart—it was twice the normal size. The one ray of hope amid this was my electro physicist stating the electrical activity of my heart was normal.

My thoughts broke off as Manasi stirred beside me. My mind focussed on the present, on the crickets chirping loudly outside as the digital alarm clock on the side table glowed. It read 3:03. My racing heart had calmed by now, I realised. The beads of sweat had evaporated. I shook my head in disbelief, almost. As Dr Sheth had said, no one really knew how and when would my recovery be complete. If it ever will be complete. I couldn't fall asleep and my mind raced back to the Thanksgiving break.

Bhushan, Priya and Siya had driven down from Austin to spend the holiday with us. The house came alive with laughter and banter. While I did not have dietary restrictions initially, the last consultation with the doctor made me aware I needed a renewed focus on exercise and diet. My stats had to improve within the next two months. Amid all the family fun, I attempted to surprise Vivi. My body felt fine and limber so I took a ball and called out, 'Vivi, come outside.' Everyone turned in surprise, and Vivi's reaction said it all—he could not believe the moment was happening.

Recalling the memory, I chuckled. It had been special indeed. I managed to feebly kick the ball around for a bit as everyone cheered us on from the sidelines. Vivi ran amok, running circles around me, happy to share this special moment. I couldn't play much, but I felt relieved after—I had kept my promise.

Every day was a battle, it still is. One needs to take heart from small victories. While my kidneys and other internal organs had recovered, I still had work cut out to improve my cognitive functions. My next check-up, in December, was vindication. The weeks of renewed vigour in terms of exercises projected my lung capacity at 40 per cent. My EF was within 35-40 per cent, leaning heavily towards the higher number. Prior to the actual meeting with Dr Sheth, Manasi would anxiously wait outside as I underwent ultrasounds. She would keep praying the entire time I was inside. This time, the doctor met with her when I was still undergoing scans. 'Rohan's heart looks so much better than in October,' he informed her, as Manasi released a breath of relief. Whatever we were doing at home was working.

I think that result was the push I needed. After an indulgent winter break with the full family, I pushed myself in the first month of the new year. The world was still chaotic but I could do my part in keeping my loved ones close. And, the official approval given to vaccines and their subsequent rollout had raised our hopes. I began to add short jogs to my long walks. The first run was painful, leaving me breathless, but in a matter of days I felt normal. I kept increasing the yardage every second day, and also added yoga to my exercise routine. Work pressures had begun to increase and I just had to keep myself fit. So, I reached out to my physician-cousin at the Harvard Medical School. Her advice was to get sound sleep, drink fluids and discipline my eating habits.

Just some weeks before Manasi and I were scheduled to take our first vaccine shots, Texas underwent a natural calamity. A freak winter storm spread havoc—power grid outages, record-low temperatures, icy roads and deaths— all over the state. We lost power, too, and our house was plunged into darkness amid the freezing temperature for a while. I was worried for my family's safety, and in all the panic I ignored myself. I failed to keep myself hydrated, failed to sleep well, failed to eat much during that week. I was constantly anxious and stressing.

It was a crucial mistake to make. The week-long disruption in my recovery routine led to chest pains and an increase in my heart rate. That resulted in sudden shortness of breath. Like always, I have to be thankful for Manasi's sixth sense. It was because of her coercion that I went to the emergency room for a check-up. I was advised to get admitted to a hospital. I have been in hospitals far too many times than I care to remember, and my last visit was deadly. I did not care to revisit the memory I was trying so hard to erase. However, Manasi kept insisting, so I finally checked myself in at the nearby hospital. I won't lie, it was terrifying. I tried to keep a brave face for the children when we spoke over video. I tossed and turned that entire night.

My tests came back normal the next morning. I can't explain the relief that washed over me. I think I was holding my breath unintentionally until I heard the nurse's words. 'Dehydration and stress,' they insisted, and I understood how fatal it could have been. It was a hard lesson to learn, that I still had miles to go in my recovery process.

I pushed forward in earnest. I was regaining some of my body weight, my legs were strengthening, I was driving properly, I was playing with my children without getting tired—and after our vaccine shots, our minds felt relieved. It was a reprieve, of sorts, amid the global gloom.

By the time I went back for another check-up in April, Manasi and I could not contain our glee at my numbers. My EF had gone up to around 50 per cent (a healthy human's normal range is 50-70), and my lung capacity had increased to 41.2 per cent. My blood thinner and nerve pain medication were drastically reduced while I was now easily jogging over 400 yards consistently every day. Every small victory seemed like a miracle. I hoped to keep it up until the next visit in October. I could hear the joy in my parents' voices when I told them the good news. Manasi's parents sent a special prayer to the gods to thank them for keeping me safe.

As I sat and mulled over the year, dawn had broken. The crickets were long gone. The clock showed it was almost 5.30 am. I was so wrapped up in my thoughts that I had not noticed Manasi waking up. It was only when her touch jolted me, that I realised there was concern on her face. She was worried I was not okay.

'Everything's fine,' I smiled to reassure her. 'I was just thinking about the day ahead. I promised the twins and Vivi that I would take them to the park.'

'Listen, you can't exert yourself, okay? Please...' Manasi pleaded.

My recovery has been a seesaw, but it has improved considerably since the time I woke up in a hospital bed over a year ago. It may take me years to fully recover, or maybe, that will never happen. I have to be open to all possibilities. All I want is to stay healthy and fit and spend every second with my family close to me. I can never take anything for granted, ever again.

Acknowledgements

We are grateful to our parents – Dilip and Rekha Bavadekar and Suhas and Madhuri Gokhale and our kids Vivaan, Ayaan and Aria – for their prayers and love. We wouldn't be here if not for their strength that helped us hope amid all the uncertainty.

We would like to thank our co-author, Sharmistha Chaudhuri, for her efforts in penning down our story so beautifully. This book would not have been possible without Dwarkanath Sanzgiri who first blogged about Rohan's hospitalization. It was him who encouraged us to write this book. Renowned sports journalist Vijay Lokapally, moved by our story, guided us in bringing our efforts to fruition. We are proud to call them our friends and will forever be grateful for their support. Thank you to Renu Kaul and her team at Vitasta for publishing our story.

Sometimes when you least expect it, good things happen. We don't know if our case falls into the 'good' category but we know Rohan would not be alive today had two complete strangers not donated their plasma to save his life. We are touched that thousands and thousands of people reached out to us, willing to help a family in distress without knowing us. Family, friends (from our school and college days in India and in the USA), current and former colleagues, donors, strangers, well-wishers, and everyone who supported our GoFundMe campaign, we are extremely grateful for every penny. We don't have words to express how indebted we are to you.

To our immediate and extended families around the world, we needed every ounce of support that you gave us. To Milind Vaze and Aditi Nerurkar, you went above and beyond in our time of need. A special thanks to our close friend Lokesh Vegi for helping when we were at our most vulnerable.

To Rohan's employer, Anthem Inc, who stood behind us like a rock. In all the uncertainty, you took care of all formalities and acknowledged the struggle we were going through, making it easier for Rohan to get the best possible treatment in a timely manner. To all of Rohan's colleagues, managers, and superiors, we are grateful for all the prayers and support you offered, and how you helped him ease back into work once he was better. We are also thankful to Dr Cristin Dickerson, Stephen Swope, Catherine Dickerson and the entire Green Imaging organization for helping Manasi fight this battle without having to worry about work.

To all the doctors, nurses, therapists, paramedics and medical staff at Baylor St. Luke's Medical Center, Kindred

Hospital and TIRR Memorial Hermann (medical center location), we thank you from the bottom of our hearts for everything you did to help Rohan recover. We must mention the efforts of Dr H Abdin, the paramedics and nurses who helped move Rohan to St. Luke's, giving him a chance at life. The chances of survival were extremely low, but with your help, Rohan beat the odds. And to the staff at HCA Pearland ER, thank you for taking great care of Rohan.

We are indebted to Dr Kalpalatha Guntupalli, who started the ball rolling; Dr Subhasis Chatterjee for accepting Rohan's case; Dr Samar Sheth, who refused to give up; Dr Joggy George who took the utmost care; Dr Michele Loor, Dr Galina Toneva, Dr. Cesar Castillo, Dr Prasad Manian, Dr Lekshmi Nair for all the care, advice and support; and Priyanka Kotian, who helped with Rohan's physiotherapy and strength recovery after he came home. We couldn't have gone through the months without the guidance from Dr Bindu Akkanti, a close family friend. We came to rely on her advice and expertise at every crucial juncture.

To Kalyani and Krishna Giri, we couldn't have survived had it not been for your support in every way possible. You have always gone above and beyond whenever a need has arisen. Thank you.

To Kala aunty, Shekar uncle and our friends from Shadow Creek Ranch community for all the nourishment and care you provided, to all the community organizations, groups and individuals in the Houston area who did their part in our journey, to Sandesh and Snehal Ghumare for aiding in our plasma hunt, to Madan Luthra of SEWA International for standing by us, and to Devi Sirigiri and the Sneha Hastam family for ensuring we never slept hungry—thank you so very much for everything.

We are thankful to Kimberly and Jessica for taking care of our children when Manasi was busy taking care of Rohan.

To Vivaan, Ayaan and Aria's teachers, thank you for being supportive and constantly checking on us. To the pediatricians, we are grateful for your valuable inputs and advise during the time the children tested positive for coronavirus.

This journey would not have been possible without the prayers and positive healings from Vasanti Gadgil, Sudha Joshi, Vidya Gadgil, Maithili Paranjape, Ravi Karmarkar, Avinash Gawade, Bharat Mehta, our family priest Jayant Joshi and Astrologers Dr Girish Date and Vasant Bhat. Thank you to Siva Sir (Prana Violet Healing) for supporting Manasi, and helping us stay positive through the tough months.

Bhushan. We don't have enough words to show how much we care, and how thankful we are for having you by our side. Right from the ambulance ride, you threw yourself into helping Rohan in any way you could—from attending meetings with medical professionals to answering calls at any time of the day from potential plasma donors, from weekly drives to Houston to check on Manasi to keeping our families updated with all developments—you did everything possible. Despite it all taking a toll on you, you never let it affect your near and dear ones. Bhushan's wife Priya and daughter Siya were always by our side, helping us at every step of the way. We have always been close to Bhushan, Priya and Siya, but this experience has brought us even closer (if that is even possible!). We love you so much.

A big thank you to each and every one of you who silently prayed and fought for us. We are overwhelmed by the love and support showered on us.

To the divine almighty, we wouldn't have survived this ordeal had YOU not been by our side and guided us through this time of crisis. We thank YOU from the bottom of our hearts.

About The Authors

Manasi Gokhale juggles between being a mother of three young children and working a full time job with ease. She works as Accounts Manager with a growing network of medical imaging services. Prior to that, Manasi served as Managing Editor of a pioneering South Asian publication in Houston. She holds a Masters degree in Public health as well as a Masters in Healthcare administration. Dancing is her passion and she enjoys participating in cultural events.

Rohan Bavadekar, came to the United States in 2001, graduated with a Masters in Engineering from Lamar University. He currently works as a Data Engineer in the Healthcare sector. Rohan is an avid sportsman with cricket being his first love. He likes to read and enjoys music of the 80s.

Sharmistha Chaudhuri, is an independent writer currently based in Austin, Texas. She has over a decade of experience working in India's leading media houses as an editor and journalist. Her by-lines have appeared in numerous publications including Outlook Traveller, Hindustan Times, The Telegraph, and National Geographic Traveller. When she's not planning trips, she's researching the origin story of ingredients and the socio-political commentary surrounding what we eat. This is her first book.

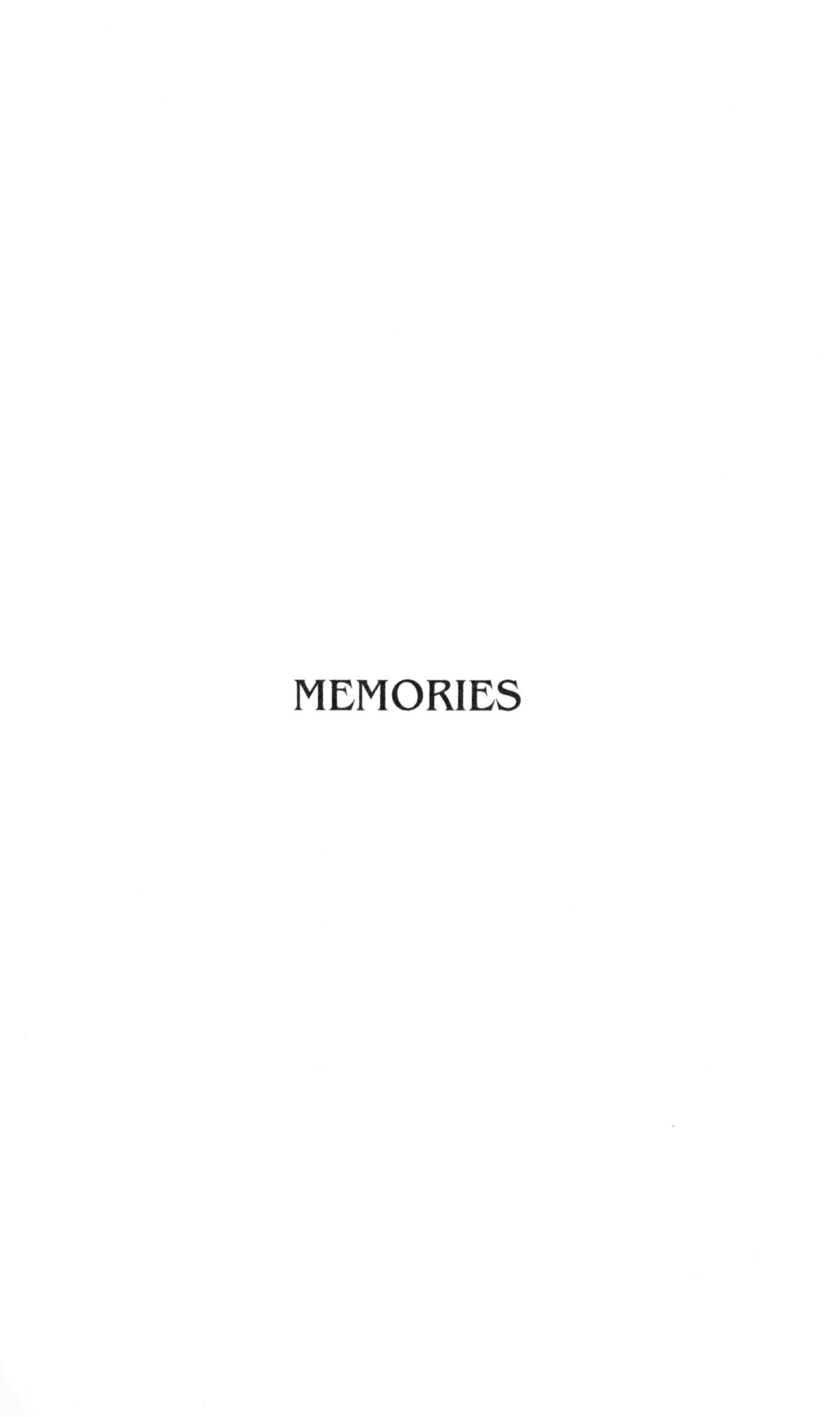

MEMORIES

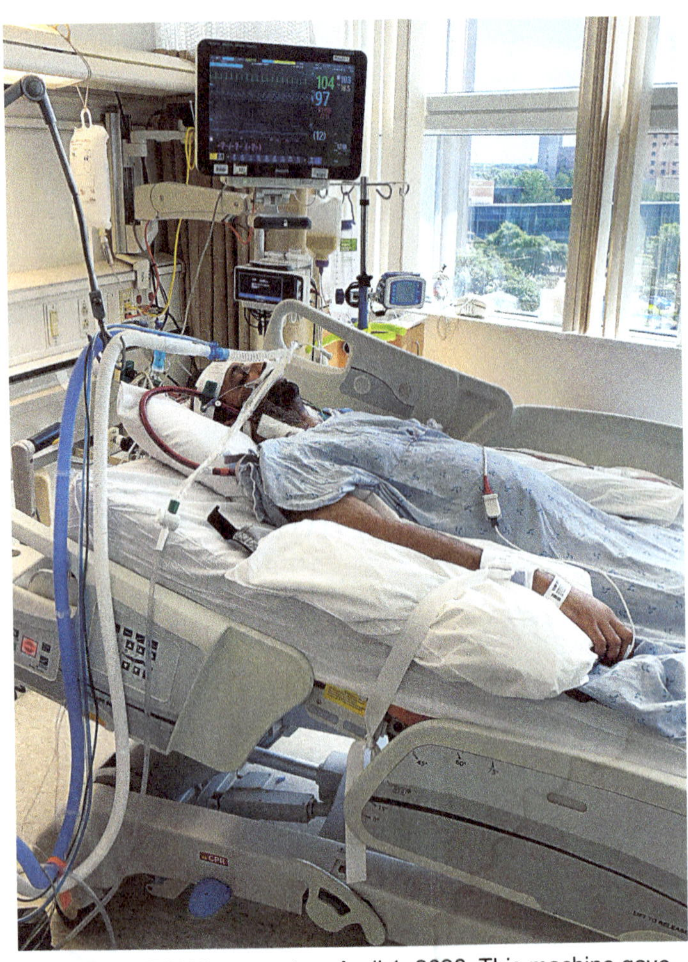

Rohan on ECMO support on April 1, 2020. This machine gave
Rohan a chance at survival.

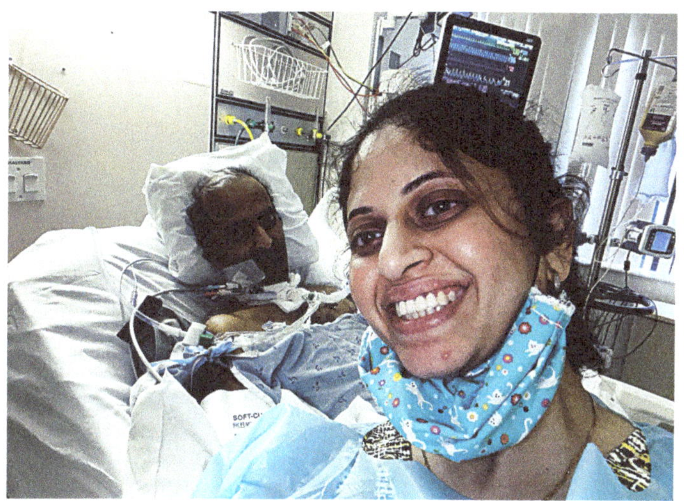

Manasi visited the hospital to meet Rohan in person for the first time on May 13, 2020.

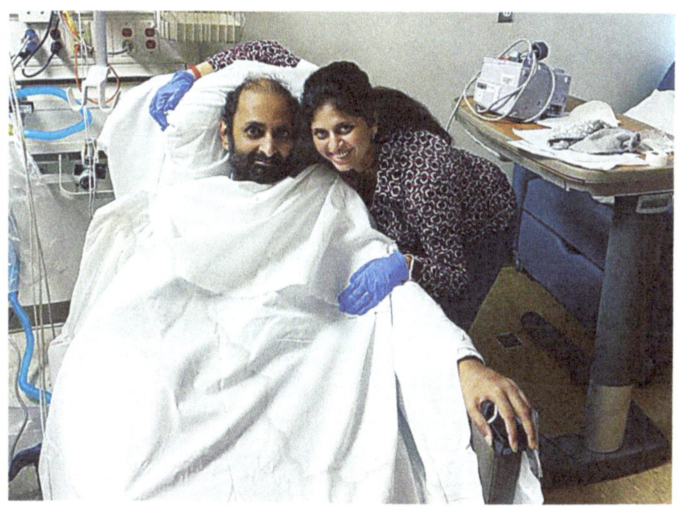

Rohan sat upright on a chair for the first time on June 1, 2020.

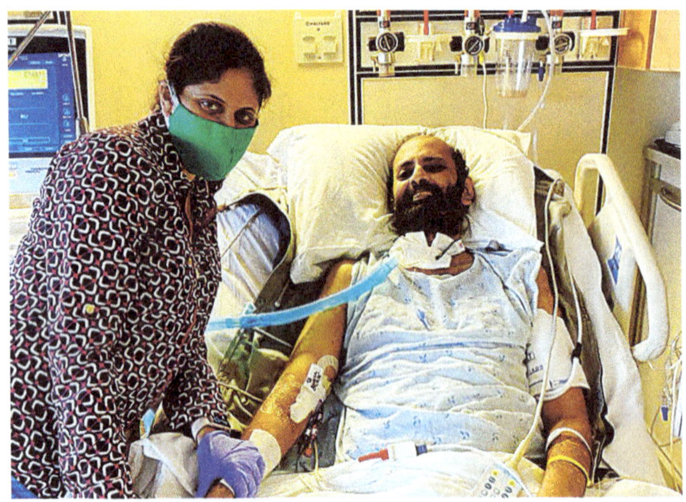

The day of the much-anticipated move to the Long Term Acute Care Hospital on June 12, 2020.

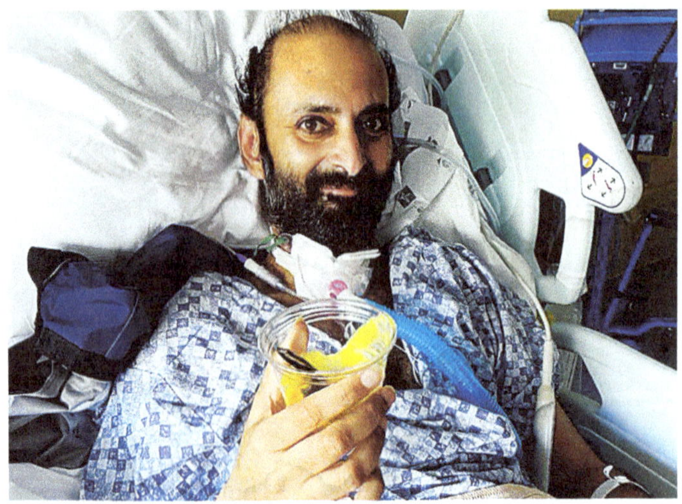

Rohan celebrated passing the swallow test with a glass of homemade mango milkshake on June 17, 2020.

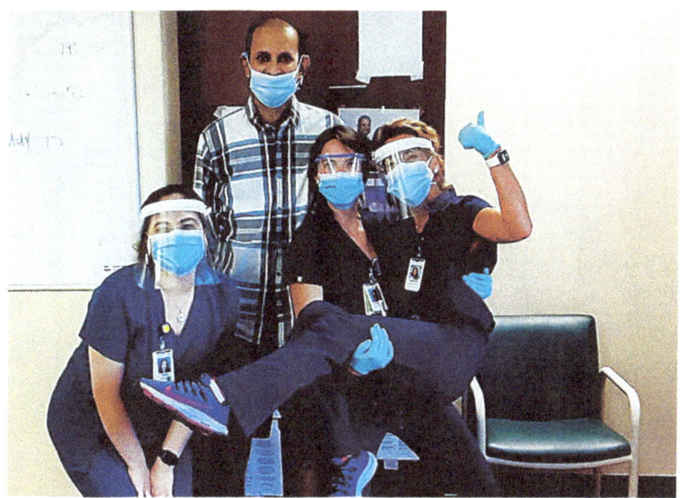

Rohan after one of his rehabilitation sessions on July 22, 2020.

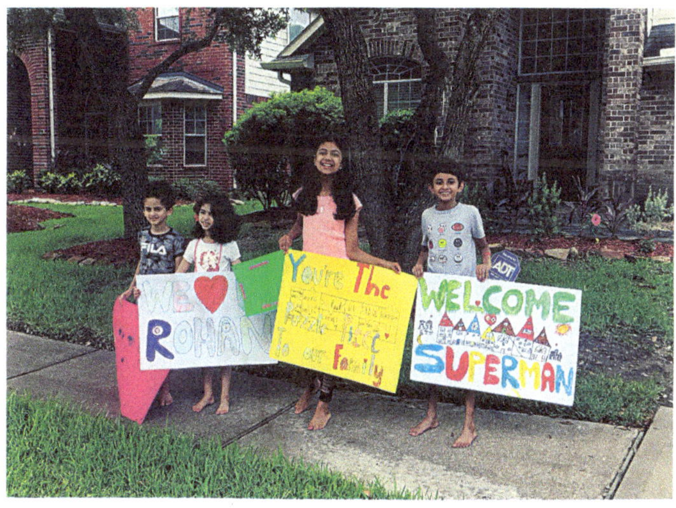

The day everyone had prayed for. The children with posters and smiles to welcome Rohan home on July 26, 2020.

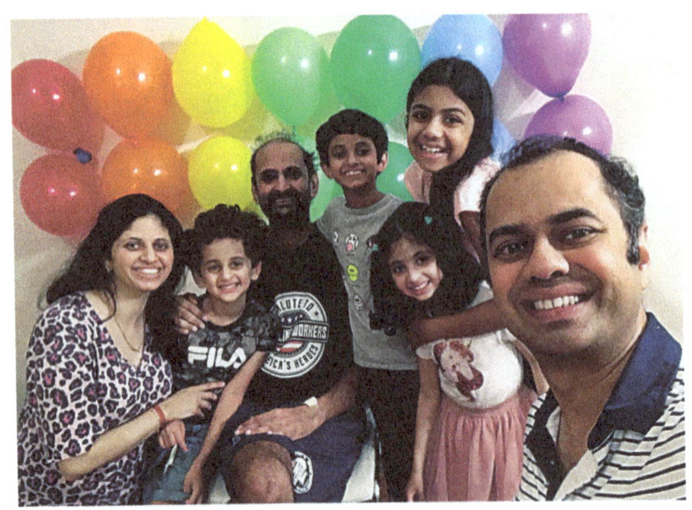

. The celebrations at home continued with smiles, pictures, hugs and Rohan's favourite foods.

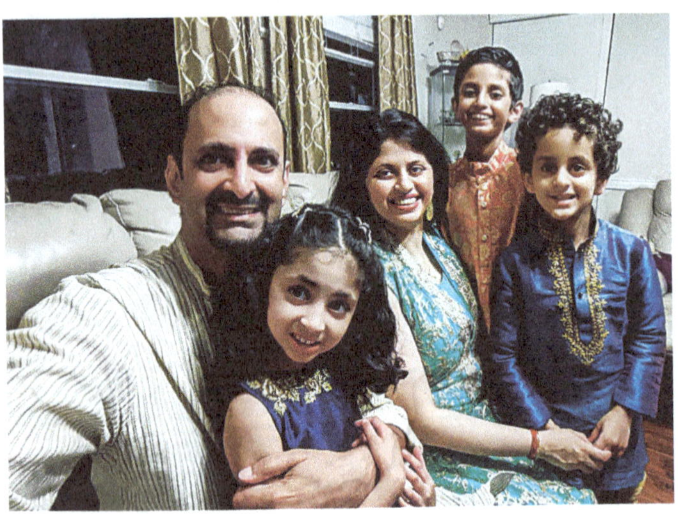

The Bavadekar-Gokhale family celebrated Diwali in 2020.

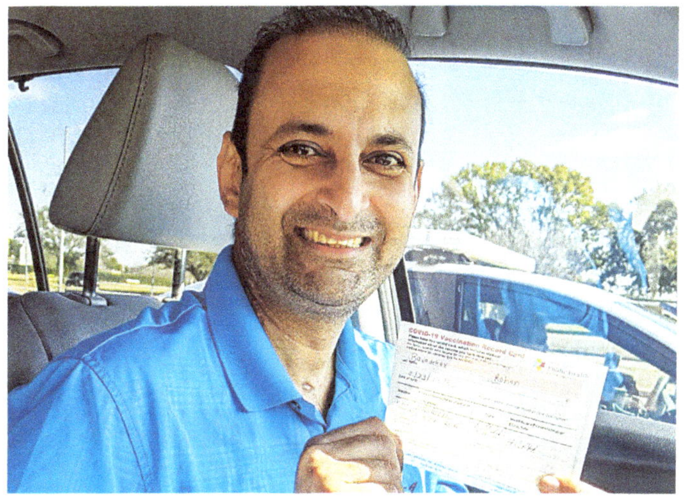

Rohan after his first vaccination dose on January 7, 2021.

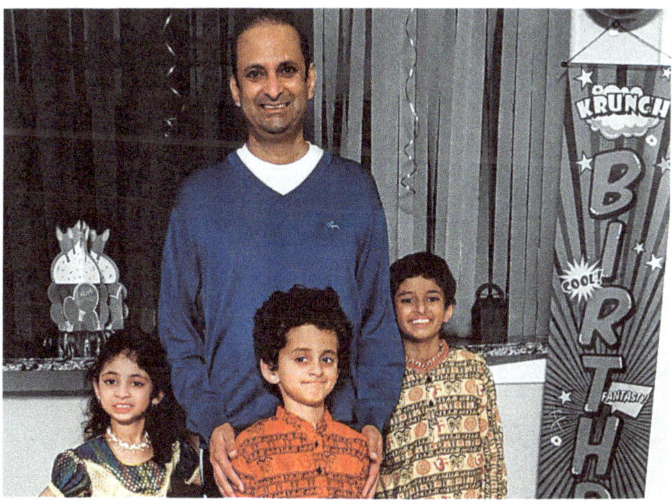

Rohan celebrated his 43rd birthday on January 23, 2021. Every birthday is special but this one was sweeter than any other.

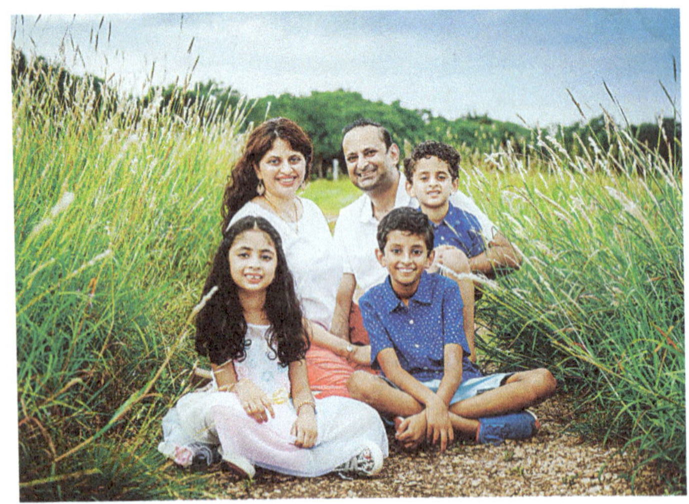

A family portrait in July 2021 to mark the anniversary of Rohan's homecoming.

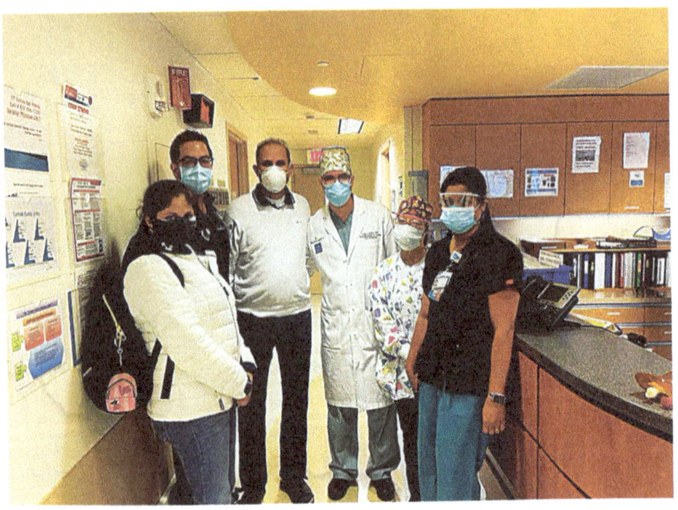

Rohan and Manasi with the cardiac ICU staff at the hospital.

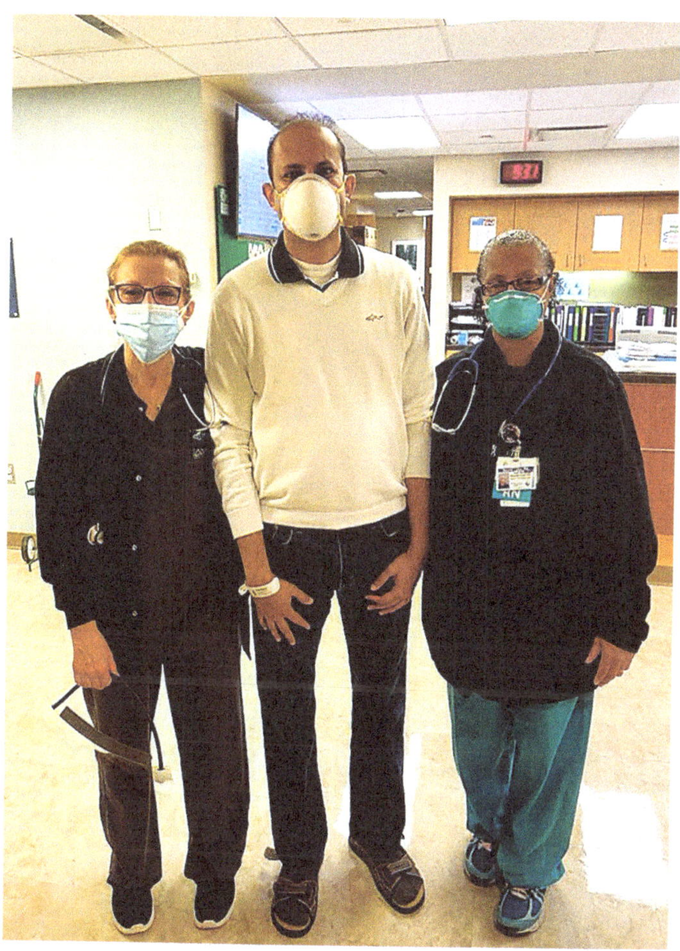

Rohan with respiratory therapist (right) and head nurse (left).